Fetal Monitoring in Practice

Fetal Monitoring in Practice

Fifth Edition

DONALD GIBB, MSC MD MRCP FRCOG

Consultant Obstetrician and Gynaecologist
Director of The Birth Company with The Portland Hospital, London, UK;
Previously Director of Women's Services
King's College Hospital, London, UK

SABARATNAM ARULKUMARAN, KB PhD DSc FRCS FRCOG

Professor Emeritus of Obstetrics and Gynaecology
St George's University of London, London, UK;
Foundation Professor of Obstetrics and Gynaecology
University of Nicosia, Cyprus;
Visiting Professor
Institute of Global Health Policy Innovation
Imperial College, London, UK

ELSEVIER

First edition 1992
Second edition 1997
Third edition 2008
Fourth edition 2017
Fifth edition 2024

Notices

Practitioners and researchers must always rely on their own experience and knowledge in evaluating and using any information, methods, compounds or experiments described herein. Because of rapid advances in the medical sciences, in particular, independent verification of diagnoses and drug dosages should be made. To the fullest extent of the law, no responsibility is assumed by Elsevier, authors, editors or contributors for any injury and/or damage to persons or property as a matter of products liability, negligence or otherwise, or from any use or operation of any methods, products, instructions, or ideas contained in the material herein.

ISBN: 978-0-323-93145-8

Content Strategist: Andrae Akeh
Content Project Manager: Abdus Salam Mazumder
Design: Patrick C. Ferguson
Marketing Manager: Belinda Tudin

Printed in India

Last digit is the print number: 9 8 7 6 5 4 3 2 1

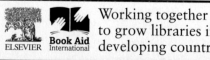

CONTENTS

FOREWORD

I am delighted to provide a foreword for this excellent and practical book edited by two experts who have long recognised that the introduction of technologies such as electronic fetal monitoring need to be supported by education and training to promote safe care and outcomes. Professor Sabaratnam Arulkumaran and Dr. Donald Gibb published their first edition in 1992 when it soon became an almost ubiquitous handbook for maternity professionals globally. This latest edition has the same passion, practical focus and accessability as the first edition, along with impressive updates from internationally recognised contributors.

This book covers every aspect of fetal monitoring: starting with a historical perspective, interpretation, and application of fetal monitoring in practice, as well as medicolegal aspects. The book is very practical with clinical scenarios in cardiotocographic interpretation, highlighting the importance of interpreting fetal heart monitoring in the context of the whole clinical picture. Emphasis is placed on holistic care highlighting the importance of risk assessment during pregnancy, at the start of labour and revisiting risk factors during labour to ensure that women have the right care in the right place for the safest outcome for them and their baby. There are excellent chapters on team communication, human factors, and best practice in education and training.

There is also a chapter by the Avoiding Brain Injury in Childbirth (ABC) Collaboration (Royal College of Obstetricians and Gynaecologists, the Royal College of Midwives and The Healthcare Improvement Studies [THIS] Institute) who have been commissioned to provide a standardised approach to fetal monitoring that has been co-designed with maternity staff, women and their birth partners. We look forward to the implementation of this excellent initiative.

This book is a must-read for maternity professionals working in intrapartum care. It will help bridge gaps in knowledge and guide us to provide safe, effective, and timely care.

RANEE THAKAR, MD FRCOG
President, Royal College of Obstetricians and Gynaecologists
Department of Obstetrics & Gynaecology
Croydon University Hospital, Croydon, UK

PREFACE TO THE FIFTH EDITION

■ ■

We are immensely pleased to be asked to revise our book which was originally published 30 years ago. We would like to think that it has helped to maintain and raise standards in labour and delivery facilities throughout the world. This book has been used as course material for our seminars which we have conducted in the UK and many other countries. It has given us great satisfaction to participate in this. This effort in education and training has become local and continuous. We hope this updated material is relevant and useful.

Sadly our efforts have not come to complete fruition as the campaign for Each Baby Counts from 2017 to 2020 has not shown any significant reduction in stillbirth and babies brain damaged after labour. At the same time the numbers of cases subject to litigation and the astronomical cost of this have not been reduced. The great pain and suffering of families remain. Repeated analysis has shown the importance of human error, lack of understanding of tests of fetal wellbeing, delays in taking action and poor teamwork.

It has been suggested that the human brain is not good enough and computer-assisted decision-making is the future. That has not turned out to be the case. Neither the INFANT study, with 46,000 pregnancies that involved computer analysis of the CTG, nor the FM-ALERT study, which used computer technology to help with CTG and ECG interpretation, has shown any improvement in clinical outcomes. This then leaves us to focus on more systematic education and assessment of practitioners on a regular basis if they are to practise in delivery units. A more refined continuous assessment will help us to focus our attention on those at high risk whilst not forgetting the simple care required for those at low risk.

We should humanize technology and not let it dehumanize us. Empathy and humanity in care is the essential foundation.

We have retained most of the case examples and basic principles in interpretation as readers have found them useful. We have reviewed the FIGO and NICE guidelines and incorporated them as we now feel appropriate. We are grateful to the distinguished authors who have contributed valuable chapters for this edition of the book. We hope this book will provide the basic knowledge to assist frontline staff in the task of delivering high-quality care in different scenarios.

We write this emerging from the COVID pandemic. There is increasing evidence of babies and mothers lost directly because of COVID. There are clear implications in the deployment of staff to the front line with damage to our ability to deal with the administration necessary to document and review practice. We all hope this will pass.

This preface seems to be about looking back but now we must move forward with renewed enthusiasm and a new optimism for the future as we hand over the education, training and improvement of clinical care to a new generation.

DONALD GIBB
SABARATNAM ARULKUMARAN
DECEMBER 2022

LIST OF CONTRIBUTORS

The editor(s) would like to acknowledge and offer grateful thanks for the input of all previous editions' contributors, without whom this new edition would not have been possible.

SABARATNAM ARULKUMARAN, KB PhD DSc FRCS FRCOG
Professor Emeritus of Obstetrics and
    Gynaecology
St George's University of London, London, UK;
Foundation Professor of Obstetrics and
    Gynaecology
University of Nicosia, Nicosia, Cyprus;
Visiting Professor, Institute of Global Health Policy
    Innovation
Imperial College, London, UK

RACHNA BAHL, MD MRCOG
Supervising consultant for Avoiding Brain Injury in
    Childbirth (ABC) programme - the collaboration
    between the RCM, RCOG and THIS;
Consultant Obstetrician
University Hospitals Bristol and Weston NHS
    Foundation Trust, Bristol, UK

LOUISE DEWICK, MBBS MRCOG
O&G Clinical Research Fellow, RCOG Intrapartum
    Fetal Surveillance Fellow for ABC Nottingham
    University Hospitals, Nottingham, UK

TIM DRAYCOTT, BSc MBBS MRCOG MD
Professor of Obstetrics
University of Bristol, Bristol, UK;
Consultant Obstetrician
Southmead University Hospital, Bristol, UK;
Former Vice President
Royal College of Obstetricians and Gynaecologists,
    London, UK

DONALD GIBB BSc, MD MRCP FRCOG
Consultant Obstetrician and Gynaecologist
Director of The Birth Company with The Portland
    Hospital, London, UK;
Previously Director of Women's Services
King's College Hospital, London, UK

WENDY RANDALL, BSc MSc RGN RM
Consultant Midwife Project Lead for Avoiding
    Brain Injury in Childbirth (ABC) programme - the
    collaboration between the RCM, RCOG and THIS
London, UK

DIOGO AYRES DE CAMPOS, MD PhD FRCOG
Professor and Head of Department of Obstetrics &
    Gynaecology
Medical School – Santa Maria Hospital
University of Lisbon, Lisbon, Portugal

KOPALASUNTHARAM MUHUNTHAN, MBBS MS FRCOG
Professor and Head of Department of Obstetrics &
    Gynaecology
University of Jaffna, Jaffna, Sri Lanka

LEONIE PENNA, MBBS FRCOG
Chief Medical Officer and Consultant Obstetrician
King's College Hospital, London, UK

PHILIP J. STEER, BSc MD FRCOG
Emeritus Professor, Academic Department of
    Obstetrics and Gynaecology
Imperial College London, London, UK;
Chelsea and Westminster Hospital, London, UK

Austin Ugwumadu, PhD FRCOG
Consultant Obstetrician and Gynaecologist &
Former Director of Women's Services
St George's Hospital, London, UK;
Honorary Senior Lecturer in Obstetrics and
    Gynaecology
St George's University of London, London, UK

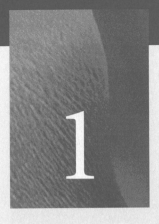

1

INTRODUCTION

DONALD GIBB

No written records of the detection of fetal life exist in western literature until the 17th century. Around 1650 Marsac, a French physician, was ridiculed in a poem by a colleague, Phillipe le Goust, for claiming to hear the heart of the fetus 'beating like the clapper of a mill'. It was not until 1818 that Francois-Isaac Mayor of Geneva, a physician, reported the fetal heart as audibly different from the maternal pulse heard by applying the ear directly to the pregnant mother's abdomen. Laënnec, a physician working in Paris around 1816, was the father of the technique of auscultation of the adult heart and lungs. Le Jumeau, Vicomte de Kergaradec (Fig. 1.1), also a physician working with Laënnec, became interested in applying this technique to other conditions including pregnancy. John Creery Ferguson, later to become first Professor of Medicine at the Queen's University of Belfast, visited Paris and met with Laënnec and Le Jumeau. On his return to Dublin in 1827, Ferguson was the first person in the British Isles to describe the fetal heart sounds. He influenced Evory Kennedy, assistant master at the Rotunda Lying-in Hospital in Dublin, who wrote his famous work entitled *Observations on Obstetric Auscultation* in 1833.[1] There was much argument over the technique of listening, some demanding the use of the stethoscope for reasons of decency only. At that time, some doctors examined pregnant women through their clothing and this respect for the modesty of the woman must have inhibited the spread of obstetric auscultation. In 1834 Anton Friedrich Hohl was the first to describe the design of the fetal stethoscope (Fig. 1.2). Depaul modified this (Fig. 1.3) describing both in his *Traite D'Auscultation Obstetricale* in 1847.[2] Although Pinard's name is most commonly associated with the stethoscope, his version followed several others, appearing only in 1876. Many papers were subsequently published in a variety of languages elaborating the technique. In 1849 Kilian proposed the 'stethoscopical indications for forceps operation' – stating that the forceps must be applied under favourable conditions without delay when the fetal heart tones diminish to less than 100 beats per minute (bpm) or when they increase to 180 bpm or when they lose their purity of tone.[3] Winkel, in 1893, empirically set the limits of the normal heart rate at 120–160 bpm. This has been carried forward for many years and reviewed in light of the large amount of material produced by electronic recording.

If hearing the fetal heart was of any value then it was recognized that this was based on a very small sample of time and subject to considerable observer variability. Listening for 15 seconds in 1 hour is to sample only 0.4% of the time. More continuous monitoring may be desirable. Technological advances in other industries set the scene for developments that led to the equipment we have today. In 1953, while working in Lewisham Hospital, southeast London, Gunn and Wood reported 'The amplification and recording of foetal heart sounds' in the *Proceedings of the Royal Society of Medicine*.[4] In 1950 Caldeyro-Barcia, in Uruguay, investigated uterine contractions scientifically with a transabdominal placement of a fluid-filled catheter independently of observations of the fetal heart which he commenced in the late 1950s.[5] In 1958, Hon pioneered electronic fetal monitoring in the USA. Caldeyro-Barcia and Hammacher in Germany

1

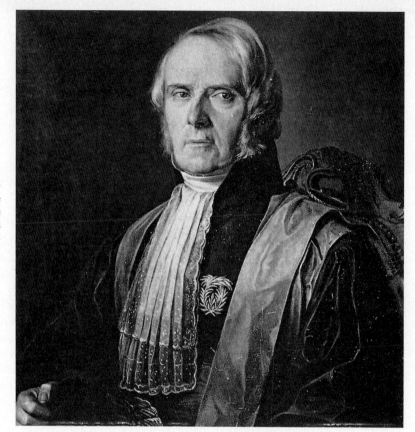

Fig. 1.1 ■ Jacques Alexandre de Kergaradec, robed as a Membre de l'Academie de Medicine Paris. (With thanks to late Professor J. H. M. Pinkerton, Emeritus Professor of Midwifery and Gynaecology, Queen's University of Belfast.)

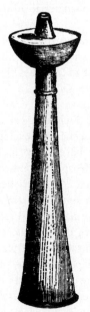

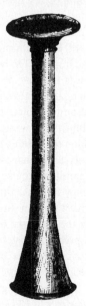

Fig. 1.2 ■ The Hohl fetal stethoscope. (Wellcome Institute Library, London.)

Fig. 1.3 ■ The Depaul fetal stethoscope. (Wellcome Institute Library, London.)

reported their observations on the various heart rate patterns associated with so-called fetal distress. This set the scene for the production of the first commercially available fetal monitor by Hammacher and Hewlett-Packard in 1968, soon to be followed by Sonicaid in the UK. It is notable that Saling in Berlin had reported the use of fetal scalp blood sampling to study fetal pH two years prior to this, in 1966.[6] Fetal scalp blood pH assessment was developed in advance of and in parallel with electronic monitoring, not as a sequel to it as might be assumed from our current practice.

The early equipment used phonocardiography, simply to listen to and record sounds coming from the maternal abdomen, as well as generating the fetal heart rate (FHR) from the fetal electrocardiograph (ECG) from a fetal scalp electrode. Phonocardiography produces inferior traces because of the other extraneous sounds that confuse the picture. This problem was solved very quickly by the introduction of Doppler ultrasound transducers. When the Doppler transducer is applied to the maternal abdomen a Doppler signal is reflected from the moving fetal heart, the location of which has already been determined by auscultation. The signal is altered by a moving structure according to the Doppler shift principle and received by the transducer in its altered form. The moving structure is usually the moving heart and the blood flowing through it. Ultrasound Doppler technology has improved considerably in recent years, and the latest generation of monitors produces excellent-quality external traces, comparable to those generated by direct ECG. The previous justification – that rupture of the membranes and application of a fetal electrode are necessary in order to generate a good-quality trace – is no longer valid. This improvement can be largely attributed to the technique of autocorrelation or dual autocorrelation and the use of wide beams. Monitoring of both twins externally has presented problems because of interference between the two Doppler beams. That has been solved in the latest equipment by the use of two different frequencies, or the same frequency but distinguished by position using ultrasound 'windows' in the two ultrasound transducers so that the beams do not interfere with each other. The direct fetal ECG can be obtained by an external or internal technique. The external technique using a number of maternal skin electrodes can provide the FHR, uterine contractions and maternal heart

rate (NICE)[7] but the fetal ECG is not adequate for ECG waveform analysis. Direct detection of the FHR from a fetal electrode applied to the fetus at vaginal examination is used in clinical practice. This is commonly called a scalp electrode but is better termed a fetal electrode in view of its possible application to the breech. All machines provide an external tocography facility through a relatively simple strain gauge transducer. It should be appreciated that this provides only an indirect assessment of the uterine contractions. It indicates the frequency and duration of contractions, but little about actual pressure or basal tone. In the unusual situation of requiring direct data about the intrauterine pressure, an intrauterine catheter is necessary with the relevant option in the machine. However, the climate of childbirth has retreated from the excessive use of invasive technology and the role of internal monitoring has become much more limited. Historically the use of a fetal scalp electrode and intrauterine pressure catheter was introduced as a package, but they address separate although sometimes linked clinical situations. Neither were assessed by the rigour of randomized controlled trials at introduction as would be mandated today. Even less were the skills required in their use systematically taught.

The clinical needs should be assessed and the specification of the machine required should be determined accordingly. A monitor to be used for antenatal monitoring does not require the intrapartum options and is therefore less expensive. Most modern monitors have similar specifications. The specification of a top-of-the-range intrapartum monitor is shown in Box 1.1.

Some hospitals have introduced electronic monitors including ECG waveform analysis (STAN technique). It is essential that staff using them should be fully trained in the technique. This is a challenge in busy units with high turnover of staff. According to the latest Cochrane review of this technology, it has reduced the need for fetal scalp blood sampling and assisted vaginal deliveries but has not reduced the caesarean section rate or intrapartum asphyxia as assessed by the incidence of metabolic acidosis or neonatal encephalopathy.[8]

Antepartum monitors are smaller and less costly. Monitors used for antenatal assessment need not have all the specifications of an intrapartum monitor. There is some evidence that a computerized interpretation system may assist in antenatal assessment, that is, using Dawes-Redman criteria.[9] Even if this is the case, we should not give up on the best computer by far: the human brain!

Hand-held Doptones now include a digital and graphic display of the heart rate (Fig. 1.4). Some models are waterproof for use in the water-labour scenario. Low-cost printers that can be attached to such devices are being developed. Such systems offer exciting possibilities to countries that have not yet started on the troublesome journey of extensive electronic fetal monitoring. They must be helped to avoid the costly mistakes

---

BOX 1.1
SPECIFICATION OF INTRAPARTUM MONITOR

Reliable
User friendly with operating manual and video
Robust with customized trolley
Fetal heart rate by external Doppler ultrasound (US) with autocorrelation
Fetal heart rate by fetal electrode (ECG)
Twin monitoring US and ECG
Twin monitoring US and US
Maternal heart rate
Event marker
External tocography
Internal tocography as an option
Mode, date and time printout
Keypad as an option
Automatic blood pressure, pulse and SaO_2 facility (an option selectively for high-risk labours)

---

made by the more developed countries. Technology should be appropriate, low cost and high quality.

Telemetric transmission of the cardiotocograph (CTG) has become more practicable with improved technology in recent years, allowing the woman to remain mobile in labour. However, more selective use of the technology has meant that some of the women who had telemetric monitoring do not actually require continuous electronic monitoring. The use of mobile epidural anaesthesia and of water pools has rekindled interest in this kind of technology. It is very reassuring during a labour in water to be able to listen to and record the fetal heart after a contraction using telemetric technology. We can increase our confidence in water birth.

A solid trolley is an important investment to protect the machine during its busy life in the clinical area. Servicing, back-up and supplies of paper and electrodes must be assured. Modern machines have been factory tested to ensure proper functioning in any climate in the world. They are designed to be used 24 hours a day, seven days a week. Although the concept of rest and recovery is valid for human beings, it is not necessary for such machines! The electronic clock timings are battery dependent and require adjustment with time changes in the autumn and spring unless the machine has an automated system of 'radio clock' which synchronizes with the time change as in computers and mobile phones. CTG timings are important in record keeping.

An important step is to identify the midwifery and technical staff who will be responsible for day-to-day supervision and maintenance of this equipment. It is

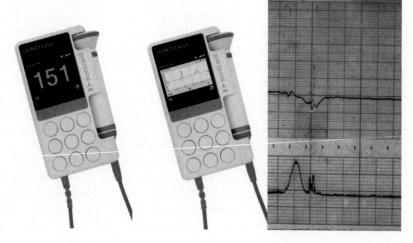

Fig. 1.4 ▪ Digital and graphic display Doppler which should be able to detect absent variability and shallow ominous decelerations.

uncommon for such equipment to develop technical faults, and defects will more often be user related. Simple housekeeping and in-service education will pay dividends. Fairly simple instructions sometimes not given due attention include not putting jelly on the tocograph transducer, not breaking the plugs by using push–pull rather than screw action, being careful that transducer cables are not run over and broken by trolley wheels, and ensuring the use of the correct paper the right way round. The less-frequent need to use a scalp electrode should not be forgotten, and these electrodes should remain readily available in the delivery area. An expensive piece of equipment requires commonsense care. It is a pity if equipment is out of action because of user errors.

REFERENCES

[1] Kennedy E. Observations on obstetric auscultation: with an analysis of the evidences of pregnancy and an inquiry into the proofs of the life and death of the foetus in utero. Dublin: Hodges and Smith; 1833. Online. Available: https://archive.org/details/observationsonob1833kenn. [accessed 10.08.16].

[2] Depaul J-A-H. Traite d'auscultation obstetricale. Paris: Labé; 1847.

[3] Kilian, quoted by Jaggard WW. In: Hirst BC, editor. A system of obstetrics. Philadelphia: Lea Broth; 1888.

[4] Gunn AL, Wood MC. The amplification and recording of fœtal heart sounds [abridged]. Proc R Soc Med 1953;46(2):85–91.

[5] Caldeyro-Barcia R, Alvarez H. Abnormal uterine action in labor. Br J Obstetrics Gynecol 1952;59:646–656.

[6] Saling E. Amnioscopy and fetal blood sampling: observations on foetal acidosis. Arch Dis Child 1966;41:472–476.

[7] Medical technology guidance scope Novii Wireless Patch system for maternal and fetal monitoring. Online. Available: https://www.nice.org.uk/guidance/gid-mt557/documents/final-scope. [accessed 01.01.2022].

[8] Fetal electrocardiogram (ECG) for fetal monitoring during labour. Online. Available: https://www.cochrane.org/CD000116/PREG_fetal-electrocardiogram-ecg-fetal-monitoring-during-labour. [accessed 01.01.2022].

[9] Antenatal cardiotocography for fetal assessment. Cochrane 2015. Online. Available: https://www.ncbi.nlm.nih.gov/pmc/articles/PMC6510058/. [accessed 01.01.22].

2

CLINICAL ASSESSMENT AND RECORDING

DONALD GIBB ■ SABARATNAM ARULKUMARAN

The journey of birth is a challenging one for any individual. We should think of the baby in the womb as an individual to be observed and examined. We must develop an appreciation of fetal life and existence. When we perform an ultrasound scan, we see the baby moving its limbs, yawning, smiling, hiccoughing and passing urine to make amniotic fluid. When we examine the mother's abdomen and listen to the fetal heart, we must think this way. What is the baby doing: is it awake or asleep, is it sick or healthy, is it happy or sad? A moving baby, a hiccoughing baby, a well-grown baby is generally healthy and happy. We must consider the reasons why the baby may not be healthy using the fetal heart pattern as contributory evidence, not as an endpoint. The process of labour and birth is a challenge for the fetus. The fetus, particularly its head and sometimes its cord, is going to be squeezed by contractions every few minutes, increasingly until birth. With every contraction, there is cessation or reduction of blood flow into the retroplacental space, thus transiently reducing the oxygen supply to the fetus. This is similar to an adult or child having their head pushed below the water when swimming every few minutes. An individual needs to be healthy with a good reserve in order to compensate for the transient reduction in oxygen. At the beginning of labour, the healthy fetus is like a child running in a field and throwing a ball. We must not allow it to become sick and damaged. Much attention has been focused recently on the number of late stillborn babies in the United Kingdom. All are tragic; some occur before labour and some during labour.

The part of the birth journey with which we are particularly concerned is that of labour and delivery. The concept of preparation is an important one, and for our purposes, we consider this journey to start with admission to the labour ward. When we prepare for a journey, we ensure that we are in good health, our vehicle is in good condition, the roads we will drive on are safe and that we have a good insurance policy. Admission to the labour ward is the time for such a review of the pregnant mother. Intrapartum events are a continuum of antenatal events. Many babies who get into difficulty during labour have already become compromised in the antenatal period, and our surveillance system must be designed to find those fetuses and ensure their safe delivery. Assessment on admission helps us to look carefully for high-risk factors that were previously undetected or new factors that have since appeared.

On admission to the labour ward, the history is summarized, taking particular note of high-risk factors. These may be young age, poor socioeconomic status, substance abuse, individuals with previous perinatal loss, previous or existing intrauterine growth restriction (IUGR), bleeding in pregnancy, diabetes mellitus, reduced fetal movements and a variety of other markers. Breech presentation and multiple pregnancies are obvious high-risk factors. Listen to the pregnant woman; in studies of stillbirth, the woman will often feel that something is wrong but complain that she has not been listened to by the staff. On examination, general features such as height, weight, blood pressure, temperature and signs of anaemia are reviewed. Before proceeding to the vaginal examination, an abdominal examination must be complete. We still miss the breech baby. Is the 'deeply engaged' head actually a breech? We hope to avoid the embarrassment of removing the mother from the water pool when the baby is found to be breech in mid-labour. The abdominal examination includes a measurement of abdominal size, an estimate of fetal size, lie, presentation and station of the presenting part. The nature of the contractions, amniotic fluid volume estimation and auscultation of the fetal heart complete this procedure. Traditionally the size of the abdomen and fetus is assessed subjectively. The value of formalizing this with an objective value has been suggested in recent years.[1] A measure of the fundosymphysis height (FSH) in centimetres (Figs 2.1 and 2.2) provides a guide to fetal size so long

as the observers have been trained in the technique.[2,3] The fundus should not be actively pushed down during the palpation, and the height from the top of the fundus (without correcting the uterus to the midline) to the upper margin of the symphysis pubis should be measured. Ideally, a blinded measurement using the blank side of a tape measure is desirable. Due attention should be paid to the possible confounding factors of obesity, polyhydramnios, fibroids or unusual physical characteristics of the mother. After 20 weeks gestation, the FSH should be equivalent to the gestational age in centimetres ±2 cm up to 36 weeks, and ±3 cm after 36 weeks. No test should be subjected to unrealistic expectations. A tape measure is cheap, available and reasonably reliable with little inter- or intraobserver variation.[4] We are not good at identifying small babies

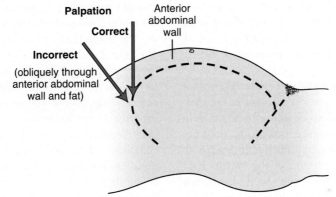

Fig. 2.1 ■ Detecting the fundus for fundosymphysis height measurement.

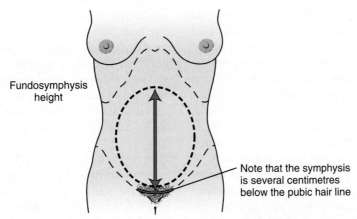

Fig. 2.2 ■ Measurement of fundosymphysis height.

in utero; this is obvious from studies of adverse perinatal outcomes. The reduced fundosymphysis height may indicate a small fetus that may be suffering from chronic asphyxia (intrauterine growth restriction; see Ch. 7). Such a fetus is more likely to develop an abnormal heart rate pattern before, and particularly during, labour. A suspicion of a large fetus is also important so that we can anticipate and prepare for mechanical problems. A history of big babies, shoulder dystocia and diabetes mellitus are all important indicators. A rewarding exercise is recording the estimated fetal weight on the partogram. With experience and regular practice, this becomes reasonably reliable. Management may be altered if abnormal labour progress becomes manifest and there is a likelihood of cephalopelvic disproportion. Marking 'beware shoulder dystocia' in the 'special features' box on the partogram of women carrying large babies, and especially those with a history of shoulder dystocia is an important preventative measure. Medical help will be organized to be readily available in the second stage of labour.

Abdominal examination is performed before vaginal examination.

A vaginal examination may be undertaken after abdominal palpation. Progressive changes in the uterine cervix permit a diagnosis of labour to be made in the presence of painful uterine contractions occurring at least once every 10 minutes (min) with or without a show or spontaneous rupture of the membranes. This is an important diagnosis. Without it, the mother should not be kept in the labour ward with the likelihood of ill-advised intervention. In this situation, the best decision is often to do nothing rather than to do something. To reduce unnecessary interventions, the World Health Organization (WHO) has introduced the labour care guide where the active phase of labour is considered after 5 cm, and more time is given for each centimetre dilatation instead of the traditional 1 cm/h. Inexperienced medical staff members sometimes seem to feel irrational pressure to intervene, which may result in an adverse outcome. Antenatal education should include an objective of the mother not admitting herself to the hospital too early in labour. Some hospitals send a midwife to perform an assessment at home. At this stage, the contractions are likely to be at least one every 5 min and are quite painful. If there has been a spontaneous rupture of the membranes without labour being present (prelabour rupture of the membranes), then a digital examination should not be performed unless a decision has already been taken to proceed to delivery. Umbilical cord compression can be excluded by running a strip of fetal heart rate (FHR) tracing without recourse to digital examination. A speculum examination may help to identify leaking amniotic fluid; however, taking relevant swabs for microbiological examination does not require speculum examination. The colour of any amniotic fluid should be recorded.

In all cases, whether labour is becoming established or not, an admission assessment of fetal health should be considered. It can be done by an 'admission cardiotocogram (CTG)' (see Ch. 8) or by 'intelligent auscultation'. The mother should be asked about her well-being, followed by that of her fetus, by enquiring about fetal movements. The last time she felt the fetal movements should be recorded. Palpation for fetal movements by the mother and midwife should be undertaken following the auscultation to determine the baseline FHR. The time at which the mother and the observer felt the fetal movements should be recorded and the opportunity taken to listen to the FHR to observe FHR acceleration. Palpation should be continued to recognize a contraction and to listen soon afterward to detect any FHR deceleration. The advantage of 'intelligent' auscultation as described is that a fetus that had accelerations can be monitored subsequently by auscultation of the FHR, as the baseline rate is likely to rise with fetal hypoxia, and decelerations may be heard soon after contractions suggesting the possibility of fetal hypoxia. The admission CTG may be of benefit if the mother did not have adequate antenatal care or one-to-one midwifery care during labour is not possible. The mother may ask, 'is my baby alright?', and this is best answered with an admission CTG. After this clinical review, a decision can be taken about the application of appropriate technology for the rest of the labour. This may consist of mobilization and intermittent monitoring by auscultation (low risk), continuous electronic monitoring (high risk) or, most commonly, a sequential combination of both. With the advance in technology, graphic display Doppler devices provide the FHR trace and can be used for intermittent auscultation, which is discussed in the next chapter. Full information should be provided to the woman and her wishes carefully considered. It should be emphasized that in every case when electronic monitoring is not being performed, then skilled, careful, intermittent auscultation is undertaken every 15 min for 1 min in the first stage and every 5 min in the second stage soon after a contraction. Should an abnormal FHR (i.e., deceleration be heard), the auscultation should be continued through the next two contractions to decide whether it is best to change the mode of surveillance to continuous electronic fetal monitoring (EFM).

All observations are then plotted on a partogram, as shown in Figure 2.3. These should be tailored to the individual case. The maternal temperature should be checked 4-hourly when the previous recording has been normal. Pulse rate and blood pressure are recorded every hour when the previous observations have been normal, with no protein detected in the urine. Abdominal palpation is recorded every 4 hours (h) prior to a vaginal examination. Each new observer should ensure the baby is not an undiagnosed breech. Expect the unexpected: breech babies are sometimes diagnosed only after the cervix has opened, and previous examiners have thought that the baby was cephalic. Urine is tested for ketones, protein and glucose whenever it is produced.

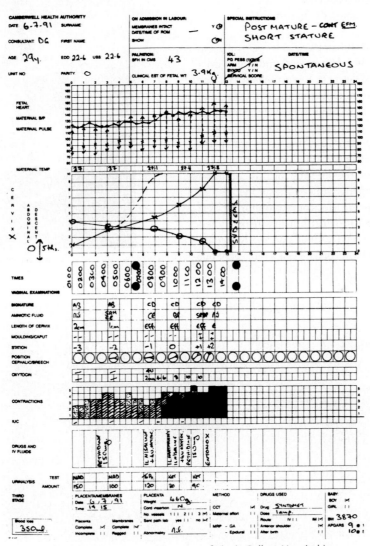

Fig. 2.3 ■ Partogram. (Courtesy of King's College Hospital.)

The programme of observations should not be rigid and will vary depending on the clinical situation.

The admission assessment is particularly important with a view to undertaking safe intermittent, limited electronic monitoring. The mother's degree of risk may change from low to high; however, indications will usually be present. A normal admission CTG in a mother who, on history and examination, is low risk assures a healthy fetus for the next 4 h unless one of four events supervenes:

1. placental abruption
2. umbilical cord prolapse
3. injudicious use of oxytocics
4. imprudent application of instruments

Placental abruption is characterized by pain, anxiety, tachycardia and often bleeding; a good midwife or doctor should suspect and detect it. It is estimated that one in five cases may have minimal or no symptoms, and the condition is diagnosed retrospectively.[5] Umbilical cord prolapse occurs after rupture of the membranes with a high presenting part. Good midwifery and medical practice should detect this early on when it occurs in the labour ward, and the outcome for this condition is excellent when properly treated. The proper use of oxytocics and appropriate electronic monitoring (see Ch. 10) and the proper use of instruments are promoted by education and training. Death of a normally formed term fetus within 4 h of a normal CTG is a rare event but certainly can occur with a serious placental abruption for which there may be no warning sign. A fetus can die of placental abruption within 15 min of a normal CTG.

The importance of clinical sense cannot be overemphasized.

Figure 2.4 shows a 'complete' CTG machine, including an accompanying tape measure and fetal stethoscope. Why is the fetal stethoscope needed? The CTG shown in Figure 2.5 was undertaken on a mother

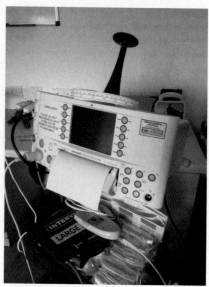

Fig. 2.4 ■ 'Complete' fetal monitor.

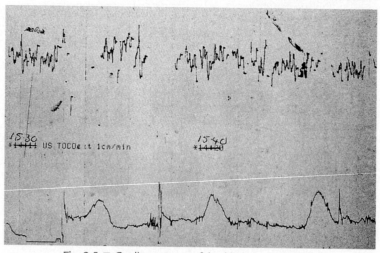

Fig. 2.5 ■ Cardiotocogram of dead baby – ultrasound.

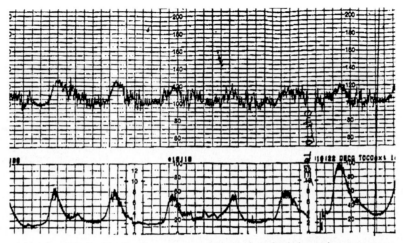

Fig. 2.6 ■ Cardiotocogram of dead baby – fetal electrode.

admitted to a hospital complaining of reduced fetal movements. The fetal stethoscope was not used, and the ultrasound transducer was applied directly to the maternal abdomen. The mother was reassured that the baby was healthy; however, a macerated stillbirth occurred 1 h later. The heart rate that had been picked up was the maternal pulse from a major vessel, the ultrasound beam having passed through the dead fetus. The mother had tachycardia on account of her anxiety. Figure 2.6 is the trace obtained when the mother was admitted to draining thick meconium, and a scalp electrode was applied with some urgency. The midwives were reassured by the trace, but the baby was born shortly thereafter as a macerated stillbirth. It was growth restricted and had died of hypoxia sometime before. On account of oligohydramnios, the fetal buttocks were in contact with the fundus, which in turn was in contact with the diaphragm, and the path of transmission of the maternal electrocardiograph (ECG) through the fetus is clear. The scalp electrode may therefore capture the maternal ECG when the fetus is dead.

The stethoscope must always be used to establish a fetal pulse different from the maternal pulse, although this advice is now superseded if the mother's heartbeat is also routinely monitored electronically. This is facilitated by modern monitors that have this ability. Some companies have introduced a mechanism that incorporates infrared sensors in the tocograph transducer ('smart pulse' – Fig. 2.7), which can detect the

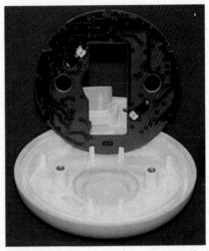

Fig. 2.7 ■ The tocographic transducer ('smart pulse'), which consists of two infrared sensors to detect superficial maternal vessel pulsations.

superficial vessel pulsations and provide a trace of the maternal heart rate (Fig. 2.8).

Figure 2.9 is the trace obtained from another mother who attended not in labour but rather complained of reduced fetal movements. The midwives applied a Hewlett-Packard 1350 fetal monitor, which included a fetal movement detector in the ultrasound transducer. The black lines in the middle of the trace indicate movements. The mother returned some hours later and delivered a macerated stillbirth. The ultrasound had again picked up the mother's pulse, but more

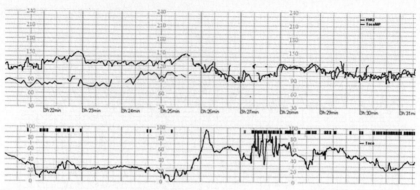

Fig. 2.8 ■ A cardiotocogram tracing that shows the maternal and fetal heart rate simultaneously using the 'smart pulse' tocographic transducer.

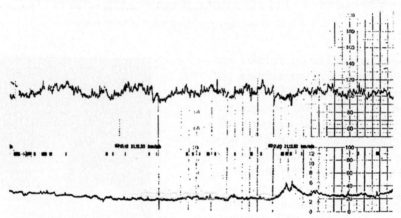

Fig. 2.9 ■ Cardiotocogram of dead baby – ultrasound with fetal movement profile.

worryingly, the movements detected were not fetal movements but the rather maternal intestinal activity or some other maternal movement. It should be noted that adult heart rate recordings also show baseline variability and accelerations. Prolonged accelerations at the time of uterine contractions and increased variability are characteristic of the maternal heart rate in the second stage when the mother has uterine contractions, and she is bearing down.[6] An increasingly recognized mistake occurs when the monitor records the maternal heart rate with accelerations (Fig. 2.10) instead of the FHR with decelerations that should be seen with head compression. This may obscure a trace that would be showing a prolonged deceleration requiring delivery. Proper clinical application and relating the FHR patterns carefully to contractions should help us to avoid these tragic pitfalls. The mother's pulse rate should be

correlated to the FHR and annotated at the beginning of the trace. The Medical Devices Agency in the UK advises that the fetal heart should be auscultated prior to the monitor being used because the maternal heart rate may be detected. The maternal heart rate may be the same as the FHR, or it may be doubled and at times increased by 50% based on the number of maternal pulses picked up and whether they are picked up continuously or intermittently.

Figure 2.11 illustrates the correct use of the 'kineto cardiotocograph' on the Hewlett-Packard 1350 monitor, showing the physiological truth of the relationship between true fetal movements and acceleration of the fetal heart rate. Figure 2.12 shows the correct use of maternal continuous heart rate recording, as is now available on all intrapartum fetal monitors, demonstrating clearly that, unsurprisingly, the adult heart shows

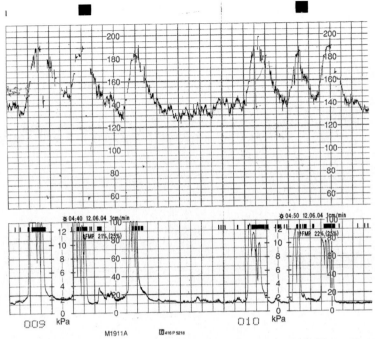

Fig. 2.10 ■ Recording in the second stage of labour – the monitor is recording the maternal heart rate, which is increasing with uterine contractions and bearing-down efforts with increased baseline variability, instead of exhibiting the typical head compression fetal heart rate decelerations.

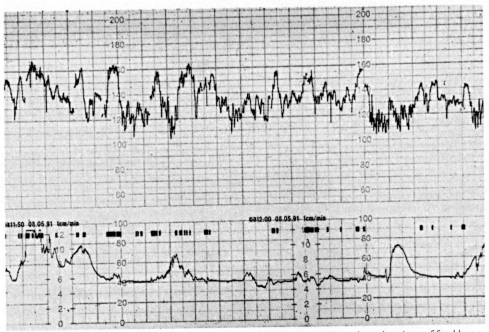

Fig. 2.11 ■ Kineto cardiotocography – relationship between fetal movements and accelerations of fetal heart rate.

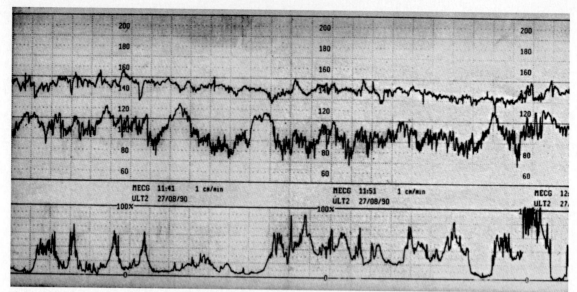

Fig. 2.12 ▪ Maternal continuous heart rate showing accelerations and good baseline variability along with fetal heart rate.

accelerations and baseline variability. Understanding this should reduce confusion in distinguishing one heart rate from the other. The use of such a facility is ideally suited but much underused in the scenario of managing preterm labour with beta-sympathomimetic therapy.

The importance of clinical sense cannot be overemphasized.

Incidentally, Figure 2.5 also shows a common day-to-day error: the incorrect setting of the clock mechanism recording the time on the trace. This may be user error, which is particularly frequent after a seasonal time change, or the batteries in the machine may be running low. It should be very simply corrected.

Good communication with the mother and her partner is vital. Obstetric cases are unique in that patients are not sick, as are those in all other departments of the hospital. On the contrary, they are experiencing one of the most important events in their lives with enormous emotional impact. The intimacy of this should not be compromised except in the 'genuine interest' of safety for mother and child. This book should help us to recognize this genuine interest. We are in a position of great privilege to assist families in one of the most important events in their lives. We must fulfill our role with diligence, care and compassion.

Our philosophy to achieve the ultimate goal of reduction in adverse birth outcomes by improving the quality of intrapartum care has been echoed by the WHO following the facility-based prospective cohort study among African women in labour – the BOLD study – Better Outcome in Labor Difficulties.[7] The purpose was also for the development of a Simplified, Effective Labor Monitoring-to-Action ('SELMA') tool.[8] The sample size was 10,000 women. This showed that whether labour progressed normally or abnormally, morbidity outcomes were seen in both groups. This study and systematic reviews on labour made the WHO conclude that in managing labour, the following should be considered:

1. **Respectful care:** Women expressed the need for supportive and respectful care during labour, including empathy and emotional support from providers;
2. **Good Communication:** Women want providers to take the time to communicate slowly and clearly with them so that they are empowered to make decisions about their care;
3. **Labour companion:** Most women would prefer to have their husband or a female relative with them because they feel lonely and scared;

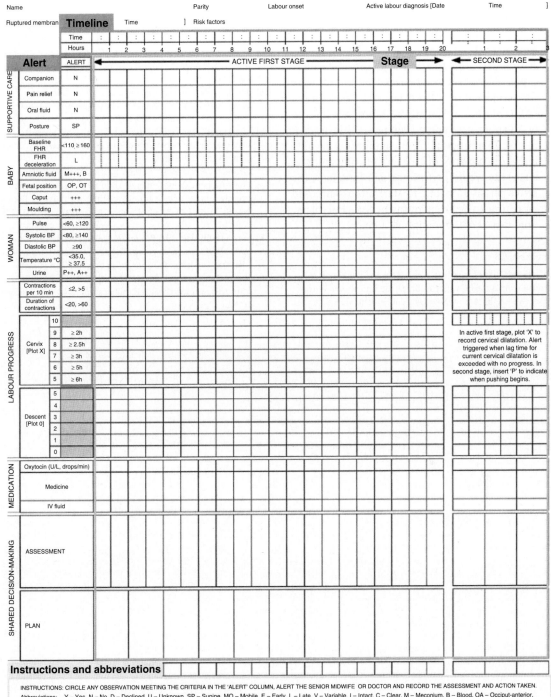

Fig. 2.13 ■ World Health Organization Labour care guide.

4. **Essential physical resources:** Women thought that hospitals were dirty, especially the patient toilets. Women described the waiting area of the hospital as overcrowded and overflowing, where women are lying on the floor waiting to be seen by providers;

5. **Actionable information system:** Providers expressed frustration when medical records were not completed in a timely fashion. Based on the BOLD studies, the WHO recommends the use of a Labour care guide (Figure 2.13) instead of the WHO partograph. It encourages the recording of the presence of an effective companion at birth who would perform certain functions, the active phase of labour to start after 5 cm, and more time to be given for further cervical dilatation instead of the traditional 1 cm/h.

REFERENCES

[1] Belizan JM, Vittar J, Nardin JC, et al. Diagnosis of intrauterine growth retardation by a simple clinical method: measurement of uterine height. Am J Obstet Gynecol 1978;131:643–6.

[2] Bennet MJ. Antenatal fetal monitoring. In: Chamberlain GVP, editor. Contemporary obstetrics and gynaecology. London: Northwood Publications; 1977. p. 117–24.

[3] Boddy K, Parboosingh IJT, Shepherd WC. A schematic approach to antenatal care. Edinburgh: Edinburgh University; 1976.

[4] Calvert PJ, Crean EE, Newcombe RG, et al. Antenatal screening by measurement of symphysis–fundus height. Br Med J 1982;285:846–9.

[5] Tikkanen M, Nuutila M, Hiilesmaa V, et al. Clinical presentation and risk factors of placental abruption. Acta Obstet Gynecol Scand 2006;85:700–5.

[6] Sherman DJ, Frenkel E, Kurzweil Y, et al. Characteristics of maternal heart rate patterns during labor and delivery. Obstet Gynecol 2002;99:542–7.

[7] Oladapo OT, Souza JP, Bohren MA, et al. WHO Better Outcomes in Labour Difficulty (BOLD) project: innovating to improve quality of care around the time of childbirth. Reprod Health 2015;12:48. Available: https://doi.org/10.1186/s12978-015-0027-6.

[8] Souza JP, Oladapo OT, Bohren MA, et al., On behalf of the WHO BOLD research group. The development of a Simplified, Effective, Labour monitoring-to-Action (SELMA) tool for Better Outcomes in Labour Difficulty (BOLD). Available: https://www.researchgate.net/publication/277235567. [accessed 10 Mar 2022].

3

INTERMITTENT AUSCULTATION OF THE FETAL HEART RATE

WENDY RANDALL ■ KOPALASUNTHARAM MUHUNTHAN ■ SABARATNAM ARULKUMARAN

Modern and sophisticated systems are available to monitor the fetal heart rate (FHR) and its pattern. On a global scale, auscultation of the FHR is still an integral part of antenatal and intrapartum monitoring of a pregnant woman and is a necessary skill for carers (healthcare providers/healthcare professionals).[1]

LOCATING THE FETAL HEART RATE

Compared with the adult, the precordium is not so easily accessible on a fetus owing to the position it adopts within the uterus in which the body lies curled up on one side with the arms and legs drawn up and the head flexed. The marker location to hear the heartbeat is the back of the fetus, between the two scapulae (Fig. 3.1). An abdominal palpation following the modified Leopold's manoeuvre will determine the lie, presentation, position and attitude of the fetus, which will help the examiner to determine the location where the fetal heartbeat is best heard. If the fetal heart cannot be definitely identified, ultrasound could be used to establish the optimal location for auscultation. The fetal heartbeat produces a distinct sound comparable to a galloping horse, which has to be distinguished from the vascular soufflé produced by uterine as well as fetal vessels.

INSTRUMENTS USED FOR FETAL AUSCULTATION

The widely used instruments in current clinical practice are the Pinard stethoscope, the De Lee stethoscope and the hand-held Doppler fetal heart rate monitor.

Pinard Stethoscope

This is a modification of the tool used to listen to the adult heartbeat by Laënnec in 1816. In its current form, the Pinard stethoscope was invented in 1895 by Adolphe Pinard, a French obstetrician. It is also referred to as a 'Pinard horn' or fetoscope (Fig. 3.2). It is an inexpensive device readily available in most countries and no consumables are needed. However, compared with other instruments used for auscultation it is difficult to use in pregnant women with a raised BMI or when the woman is restless or adopts different positions as in the birthing pool scenario.

De Lee Stethoscope

The De Lee stethoscope is available in some countries and is also inexpensive (Fig. 3.3). It is equipped with a head mount. Using a De Lee stethoscope sometimes the experienced practitioner can hear the heartbeat by 16 weeks. It is easier to hear from about 20 weeks, at which time the pregnant woman can feel the baby moving.

Hand-Held Doppler Fetal Heart Rate Monitor

The hand-held ultrasound transducer uses the Doppler effect to provide an audible sound simulating the fetal heartbeat (Fig. 3.4). Auscultating the fetal heart with a Doppler device is thought to be more comfortable for the pregnant woman and it is audible to all present in the room which serves to reassure the pregnant woman and her family. The available evidence based on Cochrane suggests that there is no improvement in neonatal outcome with the use of Doppler compared

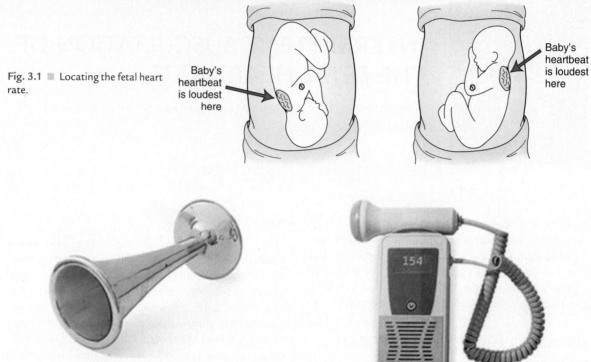

Fig. 3.1 ■ Locating the fetal heart rate.

Baby's heartbeat is loudest here

Baby's heartbeat is loudest here

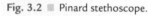

Fig. 3.2 ■ Pinard stethoscope.

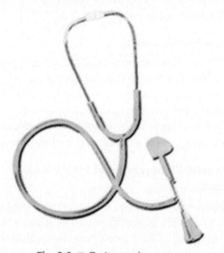

Fig. 3.3 ■ De Lee stethoscope.

Fig. 3.4 ■ Hand-held Doppler with digital display.

however, it can inadvertently pick up the maternal heart rate, which must be verified by palpating the maternal pulse simultaneously while auscultating the FHR. Although some hand-held Doppler display the FHR it is important for the practitioner to ensure that the FHR is auscultated for at least a minute immediately following a contraction and the rate assessed/ counted to ascertain the baseline FHR and assess for any decelerations or rise in baseline rate. These Doppler machines are more costly than the other two types of equipment and need batteries or charged to function. The probe is very sensitive to mechanical damage and needs careful handling.

Hand-Held Doppler Fetal Heart Rate Monitor With a Graphical Trace Display

Hand-held Doppler incorporating a small functional display screen and graphical display of the FHR have been introduced more recently (Fig. 3.5). They not only detect the FHR and display it digitally in numbers but

with intermittent auscultation (IA) by Pinard and it increases surgical interventions.[2]

The hand-held Doppler can be used in various maternal positions and locations including models suitable for use in birthing pools. Due to its sensitivity,

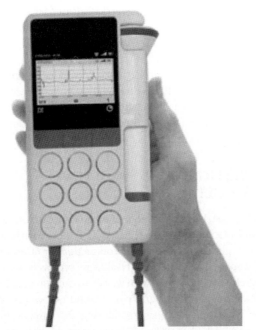

Fig. 3.5 ■ Hand-held Doppler with graphic display with storage of FHR traces.

also present the heart rate pattern as a graphical trace. The traces obtained can be annotated and stored in a microchip within the machine and can be retrieved for review or for transfer to a central unit.

This could be considered an advantage over a hand-held Doppler with only a number display as the observer can determine the baseline heart rate more accurately as well as visualize features like accelerations and decelerations. The carer will still have to have the skills to assess baseline FHR and the presence of decelerations if technology is not available. Whether the graphic display feature would improve neonatal outcome remains to be proven.

Prenatal Period

The FHR can usually be auscultated by the healthcare provider once the pregnant woman perceives fetal movements or by approximately 20 weeks of gestation, although it can be picked up from 14 weeks using a hand-held Doppler. During antenatal care for uncomplicated pregnancies, auscultation of the fetal heart may confirm that the fetus is alive but its value in predicting fetal health is low; hence, routine listening is not recommended by some sources. However, auscultation of

the fetal heart, when audible using a Doppler device, can provide reassurance to the pregnant woman and her partner.[3] It is important to discourage pregnant women from having their own Doppler device at home because failure to detect an FHR could generate potentially unnecessary anxiety or hearing an FHR may give them false reassurance stopping them from accessing care. It is safer for the pregnant woman to present to a maternity unit if they have concerns about fetal movements/their baby. If there is concern about decreased fetal movements, auscultation of the fetal heart by a healthcare professional is an important step to confirm fetus viability before further actions are taken.

INTRAPARTUM CARE

Initial Assessment

The healthcare professional should introduce themselves and gain consent to undertake a risk assessment of the pregnant woman and her baby including measurement of the symphysial fundal height, discussion of fetal movements, especially in the previous 24 hours, and auscultation of the baseline FHR. Utilizing this information, advice should be given regarding recommended method of monitoring, IA or electronic fetal monitoring and place of birth.

Auscultating the Fetal Heart Rate in Labour

The timing of undertaking IA is one of the most important aspects of assessing fetal well-being in labour. The pregnant woman should be asked, if it is not visually apparent, to let the healthcare professional know when the contraction starts. The healthcare professional should then place their hand on the pregnant woman's uterine fundus to palpate the contraction to enable immediate auscultation when the contraction passes. This enables the healthcare professional to assess how the fetus has coped with the contraction and a steady count should infer a normal baseline rate post-contraction, whereas an FHR that is recovering from a deceleration or overshooting the baseline should raise concern. Should concern be raised, the healthcare professional should auscultate for the next two or three contractions, and if decelerations persist, and are not a one-off occurrence, the pregnant woman should be transferred for continuous monitoring. The reliability of detecting these features can be improved by using the principles of 'Intelligent Intermittent Auscultation' (see below).

Low-Risk Women

There is general agreement in the professional literature that intermittent auscultation is an appropriate technique for fetal surveillance when a pregnant woman experiences a healthy pregnancy (i.e., low-risk pregnancy and labour). During the established *first stage* of labour, intermittent auscultation is recommended using either a Pinard stethoscope or Doppler ultrasound.

In the first stage of labour, intermittent auscultation is undertaken immediately after a palpated contraction for at least 1 minute (min), every 15 min, and the rate is recorded as a single figure on the partogram in addition to recording accelerations or decelerations if heard.

The maternal pulse is palpated at the time of FHR auscultation to make sure it is distinct from the FHR. Maternal pulse is counted for 1 min hourly and is recorded on the partogram. Whenever there are any concerns about the FHR (low or high rate) the maternal pulse is palpated to differentiate between the maternal and fetal heartbeats.

If intermittent auscultation indicates possible FHR abnormalities like rising baseline FHR or decelerations this is explained to the pregnant woman and continuous cardiotocography (CTG) is advised.[4] If a CTG has been started because of concerns arising from intermittent auscultation, but the trace is normal after 20 min, the method of monitoring can be reverted to intermittent auscultation unless there is a medical reason to recommend CTG continues, for example, additional intrapartum risk factors develop.

During the *second stage of labour*, intermittent auscultation of the FHR should be undertaken once every 5 min, immediately after a contraction for at least 1 min. If intermittent auscultation indicates possible FHR abnormalities during the second stage, a CTG should be recommended and could be reverted to intermittent auscultation if the trace is normal after 20 min.[5]

High-Risk Women

Evidence is lacking to develop an ideal intrapartum fetal monitoring scheme to improve perinatal outcomes in high-risk pregnancies. Practice guided by expert consensus and obstetric culture, which often originate in high-income countries, recommends admission CTG and continuous CTG in high-risk women. A substantial mismatch exists between international guidelines and what is locally achievable in low-resourced settings especially where electronic fetal monitoring is not available.[6]

In this event, intermittent auscultation should be undertaken as in low-risk women.

INTELLIGENT INTERMITTENT AUSCULTATION

In the past, there has been limited guidance on the technique of intermittent auscultation (IA) other than to auscultate immediately after the contraction for 60 seconds (s) as per NICE guidelines. Healthcare professionals have therefore adopted their own way of auscultating the FHR which may be via a variety of methods. However, with the increasing focus on monitoring the baseline FHR as a key determinant to fetal well-being, IA training has evolved in recent years to focus on baseline FHR monitoring. Programmes have been developed to enable the practitioner to check and therefore provide reassurance of the effectiveness of their technique to define the baseline heart rate (https://www.e-lfh.org.uk/programmes/intelligent-intermittent-auscultation-in-labour/). However, for those that find their current technique is inaccurate in defining the baseline heart rate, there are other techniques that can improve their accuracy and therefore the safety of their intrapartum care.

The concept of intelligent intermittent auscultation (IIA) embodies the following principles:

1. On initial assessment in labour: Identify a correct baseline rate excluding accelerations and decelerations, i.e. listening when there are no fetal movements or contractions.
2. Identifying a fetus that may become compromised in labour by listening immediately at the end of a palpated contraction to pick up what may be late decelerations where the FHR recovers to baseline rate after the contraction.
3. To detect rise in baseline rate on sequential recording of baseline FHR.
4. If rise in baseline FHR or decelerations were auscultated then listen with subsequent two or three

contractions and if abnormal observations were present, to arrange for CTG.

TECHNIQUE

Listening and counting the fetal heartbeats for 1 min, as per NICE guidelines, may provide an erroneous rate if there were accelerations or decelerations during the time of counting. Additionally listening for a shorter period and then multiplying by a factor to calculate the heart rate over 60 s may also provide erroneous readings if the counting for 10 or 15 s was not accurate as the error would be multiplied six or four times, respectively (Fig. 3.6).

Recently the concept of 'Intelligent Intermittent Auscultation' has been introduced to identify the features of accelerations and decelerations of the FHR in addition to identification of the correct baseline rate.[7] Practitioners may find it beneficial for their accuracy in technique by counting in segments of 15 s for at least a minute. They can then add the numbers together to provide a more accurate baseline heart rate. By using this method, it helps to identify possible accelerations and decelerations and is found to be a more accurate way to calculate the baseline FHR.

When developing the Health Education e-learning for healthcare module, two consultant midwives worked with OxSTaR simulation centre to produce FHR sounds from identified portions of CTG traces (Fig. 3.7A and B). The sound produced was extracted from the CTG to enable the practitioner to auscultate the FHR in simulation without having the visual representation of the CTG trace. However, the trace is available for practitioners to assess the accuracy of their technique as there is a correct answer that should be achieved. It was demonstrated in the implementation of the training that the accuracy of the rate the practitioner had at the end of the auscultation depended on the technique utilized.

In Fig 3.7A, the section in the oval shape was recorded. When considering possible techniques for auscultation, if the practitioner counts immediately following a contraction for 60 s as per NICE guideline they will get a figure of 132 beats per minute (bpm) as denoted by the line (a) on the picture. However, if they count in 15-second blocks, they will get the following numbers: 30, 28, 36, 38.

There is variation in these numbers which should trigger the practitioner to listen for longer; therefore it is important for the participant to think about what they are hearing. These numbers should prompt a longer auscultation, in this case, the numbers achieved would be 30, 28, 36, 38 (Fig 3.7A), then 31 and 28.

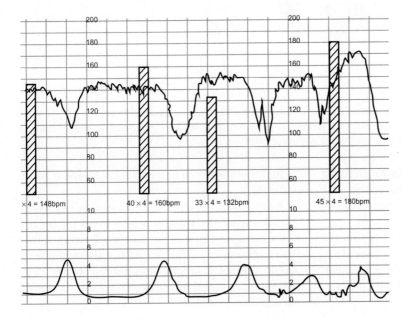

Fig. 3.6 ■ CTG shows that counting for 15 seconds and multiplying by four provides erroneous fetal heart rate as shown in the shaded bars.

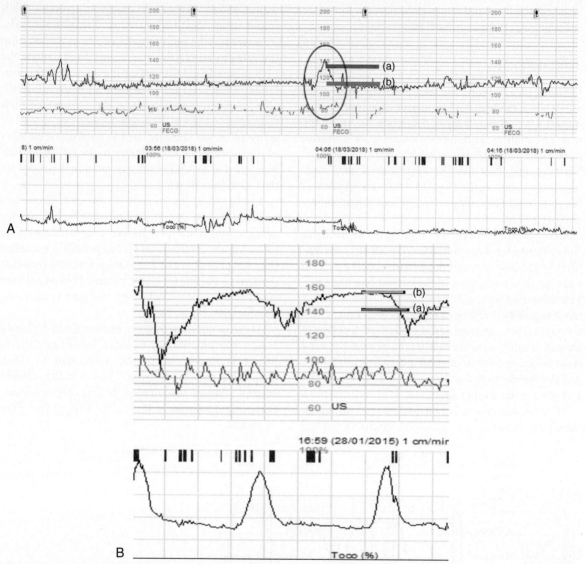

Fig. 3.7 ▧ (A) An example that detects FHR acceleration taken from the IIA e-learning for healthcare module. (B) An example that detects FHR deceleration taken from the IIA e-learning for healthcare module.

The practitioner would then be able to ascertain that the two initial numbers are similar to the final two numbers hence making up the baseline rate of 117 bpm as denoted by the line (b) in Fig 3.7B.

Getting it right is important as it could lead to over-intervention if the clinician thinks that the baseline is increasing or underintervention if they do not identify a late deceleration recovering to a higher baseline as in the Fig 3.7B.

In this example, the numbers counted would be 30, 34, 39, 41.

Again, there is variation in these numbers which should trigger the practitioner to listen for longer, again thinking about what they are hearing rather than continuous count for 60 s. These numbers should prompt a longer auscultation; in this case, the numbers would be 30, 34, 39, 41 (as previously noted), then 38 and 40.

The practitioner would then be able to ascertain that the last four numbers are similar making up the baseline rate of 158 bpm as denoted by the line (b) rather than 144 bpm if they only counted for 60 s as denoted by the line (a) (see Fig 3.7B).

ESCALATION

The previous examples clearly demonstrate the importance of getting it right and ensuring that practitioners have an accurate skill for assessing the FHR in labour and knowing which babies require additional monitoring in an obstetric unit and which babies are suitable for midwifery-led care.

While IA is aimed at the detection of FHR abnormalities with the understanding of the physiological basis of FHR variations and to revert to continuous monitoring when needed without delay, it is also important to think about the FHR in the context of other risk factors that can either be present prior to or develop during labour such as fetal growth restriction, reduced fetal movements, tachysystole, delays in labour, vaginal bleeding, meconium-stained liquor and maternal pyrexia. These should all be taken into consideration when recommending place of birth and method of fetal monitoring as the latter risk factors should prompt continuous electronic fetal monitoring on an obstetric unit.

Safety of the woman and her baby are paramount.

CONCLUSION

Fetal monitoring in labour is an important aspect of care when looking after women and their babies in labour, however, the FHR should not be seen in isolation to the wider clinical picture. Various reviews into safety in maternity care have highlighted the importance of risk assessment during pregnancy, at the start of labour and revisiting risk factors during labour to ensure that women have the right care in the right place for the safest outcome for them and their baby. Enhancing the Safety of Midwifery-led birth Enquiry (or 'ESMiE enquiry'), was set up by the Department of Health and led by the National Perinatal Epidemiology unit at the University of Oxford.[8] Its aim was to examine the care provided in cases of babies who died during or shortly after birth in midwifery-led settings or at home. Sixty-four perinatal deaths were reviewed, and although many themes echoed those highlighted by other national maternity reports, the enquiry also identified new trends unique to midwifery-led practice. Incorrect or incomplete assessment of risk was a feature in 39% of cases, and although over 70% of these cases were transferred into obstetric units, this was often delayed or enacted too late and had a direct impact on the poor outcome. Additionally, in over 50% of cases, there was also incorrect frequency or timing of IA in relation to contractions; poor, inadequate or confusing recording of IA/FHR; and failure or delay in recognizing or acting on FHR concerns. These themes were also highlighted in the recent Ockenden report and all maternity services should be focused on improving these aspects of care, especially the training on fetal surveillance in labour.[9]

Additional Information

For a webinar tutorial of intelligent auscultation, the reader is referred to:

- e-learning programme for intelligent intermittent auscultation...
- www.patientsafetyoxford.org › safety-in-maternity › e-lea...

For use of graphic display Doppler, the reader is referred to a manufacturer's site:

- Intelligent Intermittent Auscultation–Professor Sir Arulkumaran www.youtube.com ' watch

REFERENCES

1. Lewis D, Downe S. FIGO Intrapartum Fetal Monitoring Expert Consensus Panel. FIGO consensus guidelines on intrapartum fetal monitoring: intermittent auscultation. Int J Gynecol Obstet 2015;131(1):9–12.
2. Martis R, Emilia O, Nurdati DS, Brown J. What is the most effective way to listen intermittently to the baby's heart in labour to improve the baby's well-being? Cochrane 2017;(2):CD008680. https://www.cochrane.org/CD008680/PREG_what-most-effective-way-listen-intermittently-babys-heart-labour-improve-babys-well-being.
3. National Institute for Health and Clinical Excellence (NICE). Antenatal care NICE guideline. Published: August 2021. www.nice.org.uk/guidance/ng201 (accessed 12 December 2022).
4. National Institute for Health and Clinical Excellence (NICE). Intrapartum care for healthy women and babies NICE guideline. Published: December 2014. Last updated February 2017.

5. National Institute for Health and Clinical Excellence (NICE). Intrapartum care for healthy women and babies NICE guideline. Published: December 2014. Last updated February 2017.

6. Housseine N, Punt MC, Browne JL, et al. Delphi consensus statement on intrapartum fetal monitoring in low-resource settings. Int J Gynaecol Obstet 2019;146(1):8–16. https://doi. org/10.1002/ijgo.12724.

7. Maude RM, Skinner JP, Foureur MJ. Intelligent structured intermittent auscultation (ISIA): evaluation of a decision-making framework for fetal heart monitoring of low-risk women. BMC Pregnancy Childbirth 2014;14:184. https://doi. org/10.1186/1471-2393-14-184.

8. Intrapartum-related perinatal deaths in births planned in midwifery-led settings in Great Britain: findings and recommendations from the ESMiE confidential enquiry (wiley.com).

9. Findings, conclusions and essential actions from the independent review of maternity services at the Shrewsbury and Telford Hospital NHS Trust. 2022. https://www. ockendenmaternityreview.org.uk/# Accessed 10.12.22.

4

ELECTRONIC FETAL MONITORING: TERMINOLOGY AND INTERPRETATION – THE BASICS

DONALD GIBB ■ SABARATNAM ARULKUMARAN

Even when we all speak one language, there remain difficulties in communication because of differing uses of terminology. This may be resolved by better understanding and consideration of terms and definitions agreed upon by the International Federation of Obstetrics and Gynaecology (FIGO) Committee on Safe Motherhood and Newborn Health. These recommendations were published in 2015 in the *International Journal of Gynecology and Obstetrics*.[1] Recently the National Institute for Health and Care Excellence (NICE) has published guidelines on fetal monitoring and these are discussed in Chapter 6.[2] Without consistency of terminology, we cannot have consistency of interpretation.

Monitoring is first of all clinical and then is complemented by technological methods. No cardiotocograph (CTG) can be interpreted without careful appraisal of the clinical situation. The following list illustrates particularly high-risk factors: pre-maturity, post-maturity, poor fetal growth, reduced fetal movements, meconium-stained amniotic fluid, bleeding in pregnancy, high blood pressure, breech presentation, multiple pregnancy and diabetes mellitus. This list could be extended indefinitely and yet would still account for only a minority of women delivering babies in most labour wards. Recognition of these factors is critical.

In the UK, we refer to antepartum CTGs and intrapartum CTGs. In the USA, antepartum CTGs are referred to as non-stress tests (NSTs). These are therefore distinguished from contraction stress tests (CSTs), where the contractions are stimulated by exogenous oxytocin. In the UK, CSTs are not performed and reliance is placed on other biophysical tests of fetal well-being. The admission test (CTG) is a natural CST using the contractions of early labour.

A fetal heart rate (FHR) tracing should be technically adequate to warrant analysis. The length of the CTG strip depends on the paper speed. In the UK and Europe, it is usually 1 cm/min, whereas in the USA it is 3 cm/min. As the pattern of the trace is dramatically altered by a change in paper speed, this can lead to confusion. It should, therefore, be standardized. A paper speed of 1 cm/min for each vertical division on the paper is 1 cm and therefore 1 min. A tracing should be annotated fully. At the beginning of the trace the mother's name, reference number and pulse rate should be recorded. Modern machines automatically annotate the time and date; however, a human being has to ensure that these are correctly set in the software and changed with seasonal time changes. The newest monitors have keypads or bar-code readers with which any other information may be recorded on the trace. It is important to relate vaginal examination, change of posture, epidural and other transient events to the FHR pattern, which could have medico-legal implications at a later date. The vertical scale on the paper is usually standardized to display between 50 and 210 beats per minute (bpm) in order for visual perception and interpretation to be consistent.

A tracing should be annotated fully.

The *baseline fetal heart rate* is the mean level of the FHR when this is stable, with accelerations and decelerations excluded. It is determined over a time period of 10 min and expressed in bpm. The rate may gradually change over time; however, for one particular period it normally remains fairly constant. NICE has defined the normal range of the baseline FHR at term as 100–160 bpm, whereas FIGO defines it as 110–160 bpm.[1,2]

Rates between 100 and 110 bpm are classified as baseline *bradycardia* and as a suspicious feature. There is little concern if it is an uncomplicated baseline brady-cardia defined as a trace that has accelerations, normal baseline variability and there are no decelerations. Close involvement in the labour ward shows us that this is a relatively frequent finding and that the outcome is excellent (Fig. 4.1). One should confirm that the recording is indeed that of the fetus by auscultation and by cross-checking with the maternal pulse. Hypoxia should be suspected if the rate is below 100 bpm.

A range between 160 and 180 bpm is called a base-line *tachycardia* and is considered a suspicious feature. The outcome is good if it is an uncomplicated baseline tachycardia with accelerations, normal baseline vari-ability and no decelerations. However, fetuses at term with a baseline heart rate of between 160 and 180 bpm should be carefully evaluated (Fig. 4.2A). A baseline rate of 150 bpm may fall within the normal range but is of major concern if the fetus had a heart rate of 120 bpm at the beginning of labour. Such a situation occurs in the late first stage and second stage of a prolonged labour when the mother is tired, dehydrated and ketotic. If corrective measures are not undertaken, the rate will rise to 165–170 bpm (Fig. 4.2B).

This represents progressive compromise and is not an ideal scenario for a difficult instrumental vagi-nal delivery. Asphyxia is more likely to develop with a baseline rate of 160 compared with 110 bpm. This statement must be qualified before 34 weeks' gestation when the baseline FHR tends to be higher and a rate of up to 160 bpm is acceptable, provided accelerations are present and baseline variability is normal. Difficul-ties with identifying the baseline are considered later in this chapter.

An *acceleration* is defined as a transient increase in heart rate of 15 bpm or more and lasting 15 sec-onds (s) or more. The recording of at least two accel-erations in a 20-min period is considered a 'reactive trace'. Accelerations are a good sign of fetal health: the fetus is responding to stimuli and displaying integrity of its mechanisms controlling the heart. Accelerations are absent in situations of no fetal movements (e.g., fetal sleep), influence of some drugs, infection and intracerebral haemorrhage – hence the need for clinical correlation with the CTG findings.

A *deceleration* is a transient episode of slowing of the fetal heart rate below the baseline level of more than 15 bpm and lasting 15 s or more. Decelerations may be greater than this but not significant when other features of the heart rate are normal. When there is a reduced baseline variability (less than 5 bpm) in a non-reactive trace, decelerations may be very signifi-cant even when they are less than 15 bpm in amplitude (see below). A deceleration immediately following an acceleration recovering within 30 s is considered normal.

Baseline variability is the degree to which the base-line varies within a particular *bandwidth*, excluding

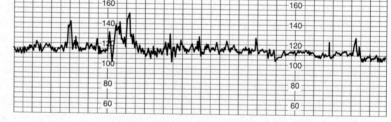

Fig. 4.1 ■ CTG – baseline fetal heart rate of 105–110 bpm.

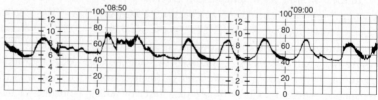

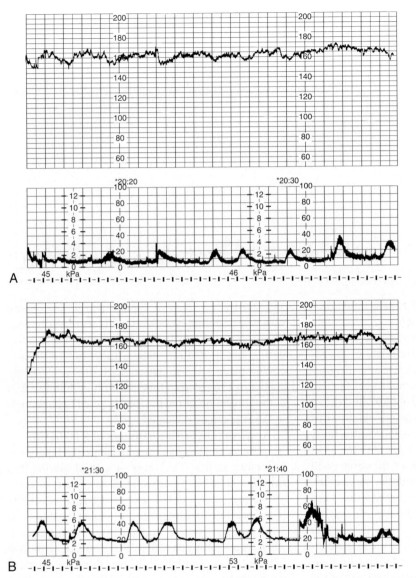

Fig. 4.2 ■ (A) Baseline rate 155–160 bpm; (B) rising to 165–170 bpm.

accelerations and decelerations (Fig. 4.3). This is a function of the oscillatory amplitude of the baseline. For the purposes of research, oscillatory frequency and oscillatory amplitude may be quantified and scored. However, this is too complex for routine clinical use and bandwidth is preferred. Figure 4.4 shows bandwidths classified as reduced (< 5 bpm), normal (5–25 bpm) and saltatory (more than 25 bpm).[1,2] The baseline variability indicates the integrity of the autonomic

nervous system. It should be assessed during a reactive period in a 1-min segment showing the greatest bandwidth. Strictly speaking, beat-to-beat variation is not seen on traces. The equipment is not designed to analyse every beat interval and it uses an averaging technique. In a 1-min interval, one cannot see 140 discrete dots. In a research situation, beat-to-beat variation can be analysed and is proportionally related to baseline variability. An understanding of the mechanism

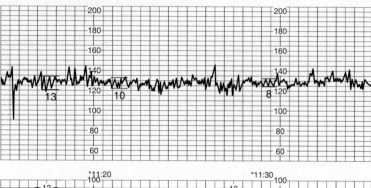

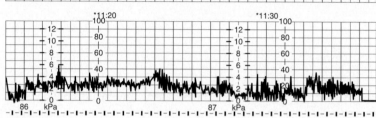

Fig. 4.3 ■ Normal bandwidth.

of production of baseline variability is crucial to an understanding of FHR interpretation.

Decelerations are *early, late* or *variable*. Early decelerations are synchronous with contractions, are usually associated with fetal head compression and therefore appear in the late first stage and second stage of labour with the descent of the head. They are usually, but not invariably, benign. Late decelerations are exactly what their name implies with respect to the contractions: onset of deceleration is greater than 20 s after the onset of contractions. As shown in Figure 4.5 the onset, nadir and recovery are all out of phase with the contraction. They are usually, but not invariably, pathological. Variable decelerations vary in shape and sometimes in timing with respect to each other. They may or may not indicate hypoxia. It is critical to evaluate the fetal condition between decelerations and its evolution with time. The integrity of the autonomic control system of the fetal heart must be evaluated (see Ch. 5).

So-called 'fetal distress', as implied from a CTG appearance, is not always indicative of hypoxia. Many fetuses are stressed and the challenge is to recognize when this progresses to hypoxic distress. Many babies are delivered operatively for 'fetal distress' (abnormal CTG) and are in excellent condition. This is the crux of the matter in considering the increased caesarean section rate after the introduction of electronic fetal monitoring. We do not *see* fetal distress on a strip of CTG paper. We *see* a FHR pattern and should describe

and classify it as such. It should then be interpreted with respect to the probability of its representing fetal compromise. Anaemia (a low haemoglobin concentration) is not treated rationally without further consideration being given to its aetiology. The same should apply to a FHR pattern that is not normal. In the light of the clinical situation, the likelihood of hypoxia and/or acidosis can be evaluated.

Accelerations are the hallmark of fetal health.

Features of a reactive trace are shown in Figure 4.6. In looking at this trace think of a child playing in a field. The child has a normal pulse rate (baseline rate), minor movements of the limbs suggestive of activity (good baseline variability) and is tossing a ball up and down (accelerations). If the child is tired or is unwell, it will start restricting its activity and stop tossing the ball (absence of accelerations is the first thing to be noticed when hypoxia develops suggesting that the child either is not well or is tired). Then the child would either sit or lie down to rest. In such a situation, it is difficult to differentiate healthy tiredness from impending sickness. A significantly raised pulse rate compared with the earlier rate after a period of rest would suggest the latter – the greater the increase more should be the concern (e.g., from 120 to 155 bpm) of significance, although it is within the range defined as normal (i.e., 110 to 160 bpm). In other words, there is more significance attached to the increase than a snapshot observation of the heart rate and considering it as normal

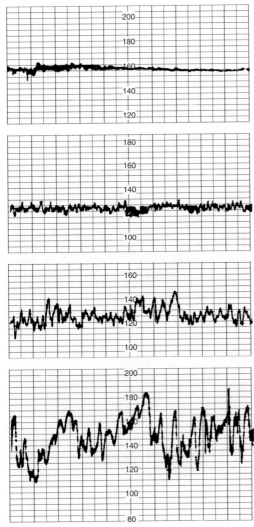

Fig. 4.4 ■ Bandwidth classification (reading downward): silent, hardly any baseline variability (not in the NICE classification, but is not a reassuring sign); reduced, <5 bpm; normal, 5–25 bpm; saltatory, over 25 bpm.

if it is within the normal range defined for observations in many babies. The fetus has limited capacity to respond to hypoxia by increasing its cardiac stroke volume and so has to increase its cardiac output by an increase in heart rate. Reduction in baseline variability and finally a flat baseline are the progressive features with increasing hypoxia. This is analogous to a rapid, thready pulse in a sick person and should be borne in mind when analysing traces. The baseline variability is due to the sympathetic and parasympathetic activities.

An injection of atropine to the mother will increase the FHR and abolish the variability owing to the abolition of the parasympathetic activity.

Figure 4.7 shows a reactive trace with accelerations, normal rate and normal variability but a section of the trace was not registered. In the segment after the missing portion there are no accelerations, a normal rate but reduced baseline variability. A child who was in good health a few minutes ago cannot suddenly become sick without an obvious reason. The absence of accelerations and reduced baseline variability suggest that the fetus is in the quiet phase. This interpretation is further strengthened because there is no increase in the baseline FHR. There are contractions present but no corresponding decelerations. This indicates that there is no stress to the fetus, such as cord compression or reduction in the retroplacental pool of blood, which may cause hypoxia. **In labour, evolution of hypoxia is 'unlikely' without decelerations**.

Figure 4.8 shows a trace with a baseline FHR of 120 bpm with normal baseline variability and an isolated deceleration followed by marked accelerations. The normal baseline rate and variability with marked accelerations (tossing the ball up and down) suggest that the fetus is not hypoxic. The isolated deceleration may be due to brief cord compression associated with fetal movement. In the intrapartum situation this may be accounted for by fetal movements, uterine contractions or reduced amniotic fluid due to the membranes having ruptured. This is not an immediate threat to the fetus, although further continuous electronic fetal monitoring is indicated. In the antenatal period, the possibility of reduced amniotic fluid has to be considered; it may be due to intrauterine growth restriction, pre-labour rupture of the membranes or prolonged pregnancy. Ultrasound evaluation should be undertaken. If the amniotic fluid volume is normal then the deceleration may be caused by pressure on the cord due to fetal movement.

Figure 4.9 shows a trace with repetitive atypical variable decelerations (deceleration starts with the onset of the contraction but recovers to the baseline rate much later than the end of the contraction). At the beginning of the trace the baseline rate is 120 bpm, there are no accelerations and the baseline variability is normal. Toward the end of the trace the baseline rate has risen to 160 bpm with a decrease in baseline

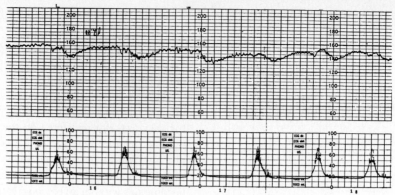

Fig. 4.5 ▓ Late deceleration.

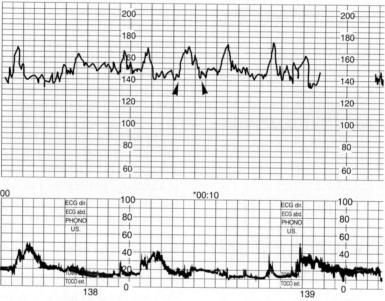

Fig. 4.6 ▓ Reactive trace – two accelerations in 20 min.

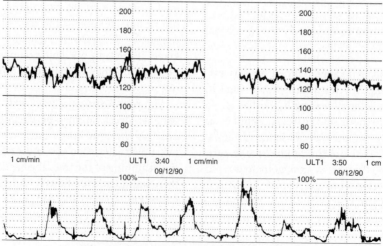

Fig. 4.7 ▓ Reactive trace with a blank section.

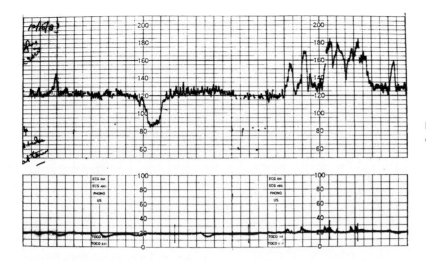

Fig. 4.8 ■ Reactive trace with isolated deceleration.

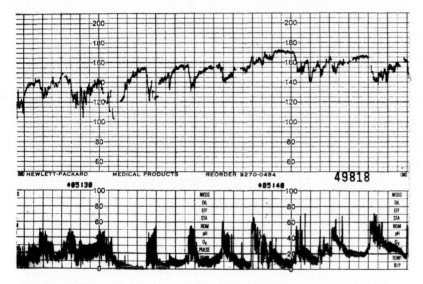

Fig. 4.9 ■ Repetitive variable decelerations – developing asphyxia.

variability. This suggests an attempt to compensate in response to the evolving hypoxia.

PAPER SPEED

It is important to check the paper speed of any CTG tracing before interpretation. It is not easy for someone who has been trained to interpret traces at 1 cm/min to then interpret a trace recorded at a speed of 3 cm/min. With current fetal monitoring technology, the paper speed is annotated automatically on the trace. If the paper speed is not annotated on the trace, scrutiny

of the contraction duration would give a clue that the paper speed is more than 1 cm/min as the contraction duration on the trace would be 2–3 min, which is an unlikely event in normal labour. Figure 4.10 shows the effect on the trace by changing paper speed during the recording. Figure 4.11 shows comparative traces recorded at different paper speeds. At the faster paper speed, features such as baseline variability, accelerations and decelerations are altered. The baseline variability appears more reduced than is actually the case, accelerations are difficult to identify (Fig. 4.11A and B), and the decelerations appear to be of a greater duration

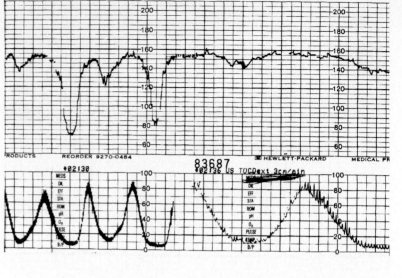

Fig. 4.10 ▓ Changing paper speed during recording.

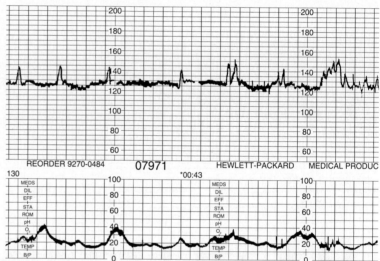

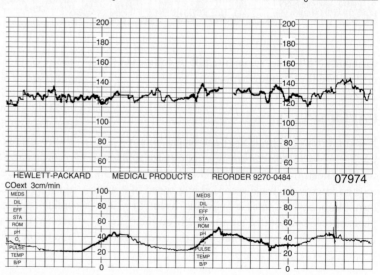

Fig. 4.11 ▓ Two recordings from the same patient at: (A) 1 cm/min; (B) 3 cm/min.

(see Fig. 4.10). To a trained eye the paper speed does not matter, but for day-to-day interpretation it is better to have the paper speed at the rate the staff is used to – failure to appreciate this has led to confusion and serious error in clinical decision-making. Current fetal monitors have the paper speed automatically annotated on the CTG paper. In addition, their paper-speed switch mechanism is either behind the paper-loading tray, which has to be removed to alter the paper speed, or in a position such that it is difficult to alter the paper speed accidently. Although the discussion on paper speed may appear trivial, failure to recognize the difference has resulted in unnecessary caesarean sections in both the antenatal and the intrapartum periods. Such simple mistakes expose the mother to an unnecessary anaesthetic and surgical risk and put her at high risk in her next pregnancy.

PROBLEMS ASSOCIATED WITH THE INTERPRETATION OF BASELINE VARIABILITY

Any FHR tracing has periods of high and low baseline variability cycles both in the antenatal and intrapartum periods. These periods of 'silent phase' with low baseline variability can be as short as 7–10 min in the antenatal period and 25–40 min in the intrapartum period.[3,4] Although baseline variability can be referred

to at any given point in the trace, the health of the baby is best judged when the trace is reactive (i.e., when the baby is active and 'playing with the ball' rather than when the baby is sleeping). It is similar to our being judged at an interview when we are active and awake rather than inactive and sleeping.

Reduced Baseline Variability

The most common reasons for reduced baseline variability are:
1. the 'sleep' or 'quiet' phase of the FHR cycle (Fig. 4.12)
2. hypoxia
3. pre-maturity
4. tachycardia (>180 bpm – due to technical issues)
5. drugs (sedatives, antihypertensives acting on the central nervous system [CNS] and anaesthetics)
6. congenital malformation (of the CNS more commonly than the cardiovascular system)
7. cardiac arrhythmias
8. fetal anaemia (Rhesus disease or fetomaternal haemorrhage)
9. fetal infection

High and Low Variability Cycles ('Cycling')

When a trace is seen with reduced baseline variability (bandwidth 5 bpm), the previous segments of the trace must be reviewed. If the preceding trace was reactive with good baseline variability, then the segment being

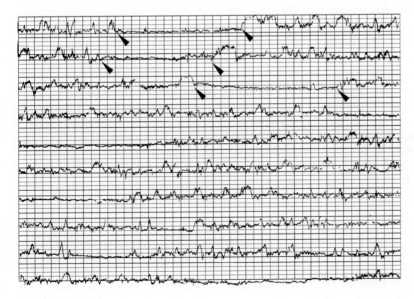

Fig. 4.12 ■ Composite trace – reduced baseline variability: period of fetal 'sleep' alternating with 'active' periods.

reviewed is probably in the 'quiet phase' of the baby's FHR cycle and there is no cause for alarm if there were no decelerations with contractions and there was no rise in baseline rate. The start of another active cycle can be awaited. Presence of decelerations and increase in the baseline rate might indicate the possibility of evolving hypoxia. If there was no previous segment of the trace to consider, the clinical picture must be reviewed to identify whether the fetus is at risk (e.g., small fundosymphysis height, post-term, thick meconium, no or scanty amniotic fluid at the time of membrane rupture, reduced fetal movements or other obstetric risk factors) or is influenced by medication (e.g., pethidine, antihypertensives, etc.) at the same time continuing the trace when reactivity with good baseline variability may appear.

Pethidine and Baseline Variability

Sometimes there is concern about giving pethidine to women in labour in case it reduces the baseline variability and obscures the reduced baseline variability of hypoxia. Before giving pethidine, it is important to ensure that the FHR trace is reactive and normal with no evidence of hypoxia. Once the pethidine is given the accelerations may not be evident and the baseline variability may become reduced as in the 'quiet' or 'sleep' phase. The period of this quiet phase following pethidine in some fetuses can extend beyond the natural quiet phase expected and thus leads to anxiety. In labour, if the trace has been reactive and the fetus was not hypoxic, hypoxia can develop only gradually owing to regular uterine contractions cutting off the blood supply to the placenta, unless acute events such as abruption, cord prolapse, scar dehiscence or oxytocic hyperstimulation occur. Alternatively, hypoxia can be caused by the reduction of blood supply to the retroplacental area due to regular uterine contractions, which will present with late decelerations, and that due to cord compression, which will present with variable decelerations. If these are affecting the fetus and causing hypoxia, the fetus tends to compensate for the hypoxia by increasing the cardiac output, which it does by increasing the FHR as it has limited capacity to increase the stroke volume. Therefore, if the FHR pattern after pethidine does not show any decelerations and there is no increase in the baseline rate, then, despite the fact that there are no

accelerations and the baseline variability is reduced, these features are likely to be due to pethidine rather than to hypoxia. When the baby is born, the baby may not cry and may need stimulation or reversal of drug effect by naloxone or assisted ventilation because of the effect of the drug on the CNS causing respiratory depression, but the neonate will have good cord arterial blood status indicating that there was no intrauterine hypoxia.

False Baseline Variability Due to Technical Reasons

Modern machines have autocorrelation and do not pose technical problems related to baseline variability, but the older machines did not possess autocorrelation and gave a false impression of exaggerated baseline variability when the FHR was recorded using an ultrasound transducer. Although one may not encounter this in current practice, traces from several years ago may be brought up to you for medico-legal reasons and hence the explanation for this problem is offered in this section.

The baseline variability seen on the trace is produced by the time differences between individual heartbeats. One segment of the serration or undulation, that is, one upswing which contributes to baseline variability, is only a few millimetres but is representative of a number of beats, as was outlined earlier. The machine calculates the beat intervals from the impulses coming back to the transducer, which arise from the movements of the fetal heart. However, there may be extraneous impulses from other sources (caused by movement of the bowel or of the anterior abdominal wall of the mother), which may be misinterpreted and a falsely exaggerated baseline variability produced (Fig. 4.13). When the fetus becomes hypoxic with progressive decelerations, usually the first feature to be observed is the disappearance of the accelerations, followed by an increase in baseline FHR, followed by a reduction in the baseline variability. Worsening of the fetal condition can be identified by progressive increase in the depth and duration of the decelerations with reduction of inter-deceleration intervals. In Figure 4.13 there is tachycardia, with an FHR of 160 bpm, there are no accelerations and there are variable decelerations suggestive of possible fetal compromise. This

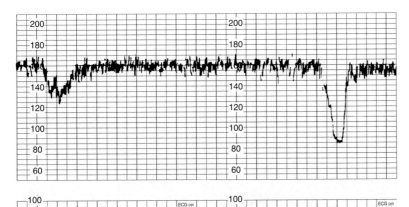

Fig. 4.13 ■ Artefactual variability due to an old machine without autocorrelation facility.

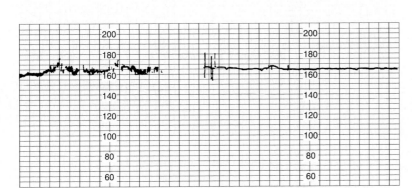

Fig. 4.14 ■ Artefactual variability obscuring pathological trace rectified by using scalp electrodes.

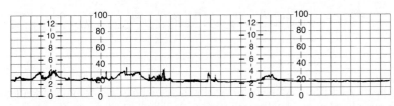

trace was from a growth-restricted fetus with little amniotic fluid surrounding it. Its other features (absence of accelerations, tachycardia and decelerations) are not consistent with the 'good baseline variability' observed on the trace. The problem is that the trace was obtained on a fetal monitor without autocorrelation facilities. The baseline variability obtained on the ultrasound mode with the old fetal monitors is not reliable and in labour it is best to use a scalp electrode with these machines. Figure 4.14

shows an abnormal trace with tachycardia, no accelerations and with reduced variability. The switch from ultrasound to direct electrocardiograph (ECG) mode gives the markedly reduced (flat) true baseline variability of the sick fetus. Use of modern machines should obviate this problem (Fig. 4.15).

Poor Contact of the Scalp Electrode

'Picket fence' artefact is not an uncommon problem with the use of scalp electrodes (Fig. 4.16). The vertical

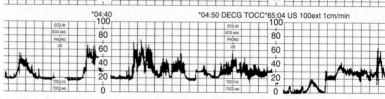

Fig. 4.15 ■ Effect on variability of changing monitoring mode from fetal electrode to ultrasound in a machine with autocorrelation facility.

Fig. 4.16 ■ 'Picket fence' artefact due to poor contact of fetal electrode.

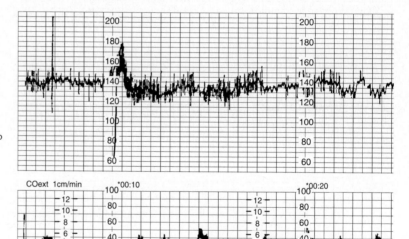

deviation of the baseline, unlike the undulations, suggests that it is an artefact. Figure 4.17 shows a baseline tachycardia with a rate of 150 bpm. There are no accelerations and careful attention reveals that the baseline variability is markedly reduced (less than 5 bpm) and is masked by artefact. This is usually thought to be due to poor contact of the electrode with fetal tissue or the absence of proper contact of the reference electrode (a metal piece at the base of the scalp electrode) with maternal tissue. Although replacing the electrode and applying an adhesive skin electrode to the maternal thigh as a reference electrode may be of

some help, usually these manoeuvres do not markedly improve the quality of the recording. In these situations, it is better to record the FHR tracing with an external ultrasound transducer that has autocorrelation facilities, as most modern equipment has. These fetal monitors give a good-quality trace with a baseline variability equivalent to that obtainable with a scalp electrode. In the past, when a good-quality trace was not obtained with external ultrasound transducers, the use of internal electrodes was advocated, whereas currently the use of external ultrasound transducers is indicated when the FHR trace with an internal

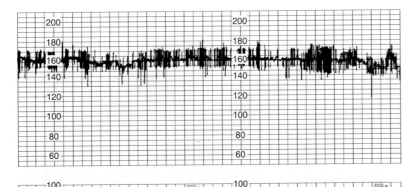

Fig. 4.17 ■ Abnormal trace with no accelerations and reduced variability being hidden by 'picket fence' artefact.

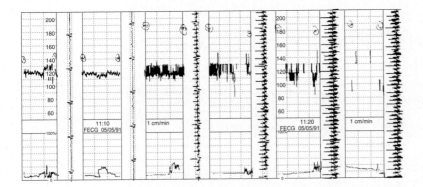

Fig. 4.18 ■ Effect of TENS on the trace as the TENS frequency rate is increased.

electrode is unsatisfactory (see Fig. 4.15). Because of the good-quality tracing obtained with fetal monitors using modern technology, there is no necessity to rupture the membranes during labour in order to place an electrode. The indications for artificial rupture of the membranes are during augmentation of slow labour and to inspect the colour of the amniotic fluid when a trace is abnormal. If the 'picket fencing' has a regular pattern and the distance above and below the baseline is nearly equal throughout the trace, then it may be due to cardiac arrhythmia. If not, it is likely to be a problem with disturbance in the signal-to-noise ratio caused by the electrode.

Other Interference

Extraneous electrical influences can produce artefact in the baseline variability; if the disturbance exceeds the frequency of signals obtained from the FHR using a scalp electrode it can completely confuse the FHR signals with no FHR tracing. The use of transcutaneous electrical nerve stimulation (TENS) or the obstetric pulsar used for pain relief can produce this problem; Figure 4.18 illustrates this with FHR tracing and the corresponding ECG signals.

With TENS, external ultrasound monitoring is preferable.

CORRECT IDENTIFICATION OF BASELINE HEART RATE

Persistent accelerations may lead to confusion such that some traces have been termed 'pseudodistress' patterns. When the fetus is very active it may show so many accelerations that it is misinterpreted as

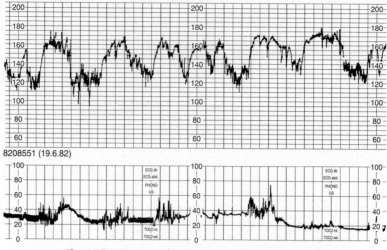

8208551 (19.6.82)

Fig. 4.19 ▪ Very reactive trace – pseudodistress pattern.

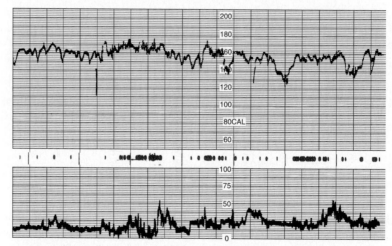

Fig. 4.20 ▪ Continuous accelerations – very frequent use of event marker.

tachycardia with decelerations (Fig. 4.19). This situation can arise in the antenatal period or during labour. Certain clues aid correct interpretation. The clinical picture and risk assessment will indicate the probability of true compromise. Figures 4.20 and 4.21 show greater degrees of the same phenomenon and are more difficult to interpret. The trace may appear to show a long period of tachycardia due to confluent accelerations. In the antenatal period, it is easier to recognize these patterns as non-pathological if the fetus is well grown, has a normal amniotic fluid volume and is moving actively during the recording of the trace. This will be most obviously demonstrated by frequent use of the event marker by the mother or by evidence of fetal movements on the tocography channel (Fig. 4.20). Many fetal monitors detect fetal movements automatically (Fig. 4.22). Such traces should have good baseline variability both at the true rate and at the higher rate. The true baseline rate on these traces is not below 110 bpm (the lower limit of normal for a healthy fetus). Inspection of the trace prior to the segment where there is doubt as to the true baseline rate would provide evidence of the true baseline rate. If such a segment is not available, continuation of the trace for a longer period should provide it. In clinical practice this pattern is repeatedly misunderstood,

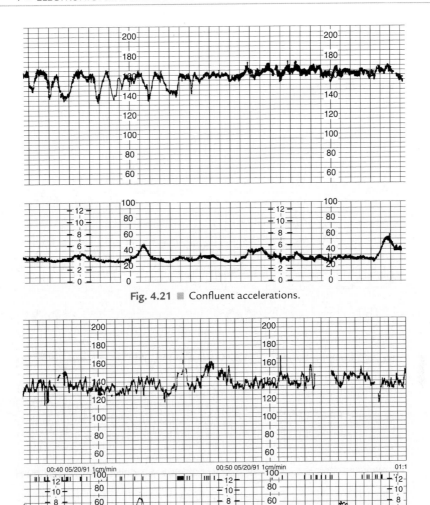

Fig. 4.21 ■ Confluent accelerations.

Fig. 4.22 ■ Hewlett-Packard 1350 with a combi transducer; automatic fetal movement recording is done through the ultrasound channel.

resulting in unnecessary intervention and the birth of a vigorous neonate behaving after delivery as it did before: Apgar scores of 9 and 10 after a caesarean section for 'fetal distress'.

A hypoxic fetus with a tachycardia with or without decelerations does not move actively.

At times, there may be difficulty in resolving this issue. Figure 4.23A may be considered to show either stress or a very active fetus. The tocography channel suggests rather frequent contractions, and after the reduction in the rate of oxytocin and contraction

frequency, a more understandable picture emerges (Fig. 4.23B). Further evaluation may be necessary with ultrasound assessment antenatally or fetal scalp blood sampling intrapartum. If an oxytocin infusion is in progress, its rate should be reduced.

Importance of Recognition of the Baseline Heart Rate for Each Fetus

When a fetus is in good health the baseline FHR tends to vary by 10–15 bpm in an undulating manner, slowing slightly in the sleep phase and after maternal sedation.

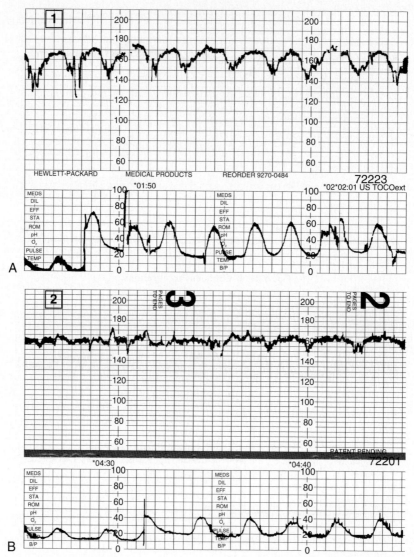

Fig. 4.23 ■ Trace showing: (A) hyperstimulation and tachycardia; (B) followed by reduction of oxytocin and resolution.

It rises slightly during the active phase when the fetus moves, exhibiting a number of accelerations. Gradually increasing hypoxia causes the FHR to rise gradually to a tachycardia. During the evolution of persistent repetitive decelerations, it is important to recognize the steadily rising baseline rate due to compensation, potentially leading to compromise. Each fetus has its own baseline rate and, although it may still be within the normal range, for that individual fetus it can represent a significant rise. It is important to take note of the baseline rate at the beginning of the trace and to compare it with the current rate. In the antenatal period, comparison of the baseline heart rate of sequential traces has the same relevance. Priority should be given to the revised definition of normal baseline FHR, 110–160 bpm, bearing these considerations in mind. Any tracing with a baseline rate of greater than 160 bpm should be carefully scrutinized for other suspicious features. Traces within the normal range for baseline rate may be abnormal or ominous on account of other features (Fig. 4.24).

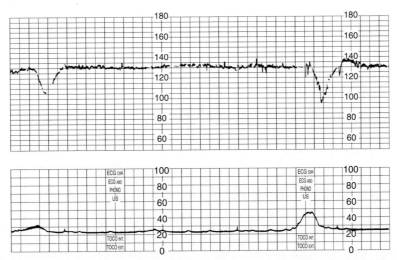

Fig. 4.24 ■ Normal baseline rate – pathological trace, with no accelerations, reduced baseline variability ('silent pattern') and shallow late decelerations.

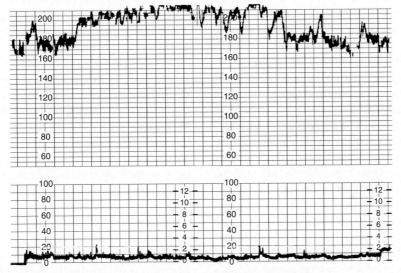

Fig. 4.25 ■ Moderate baseline tachycardia (150–170 bpm); other features are reassuring.

A normal baseline rate can be associated with hypoxia and an ominous trace.

Baseline Tachycardia and Bradycardia

A range of 160–180 bpm is termed a *baseline tachycardia* and a range of 100–110 bpm is called *baseline bradycardia*. Although they are categorized in the 'suspicious' category in various guidelines, provided there is good baseline variability, accelerations and an absence of decelerations, these FHRs do not generally represent hypoxia. Figure 4.25 shows a moderate baseline tachycardia although other features are reassuring.

Figure 4.26 is a rare trace showing sinus bradycardia at 80 bpm with a trace that is otherwise remarkably normal. The baby was born in good condition with a good outcome. The mother had had a renal transplant and was taking various medications including

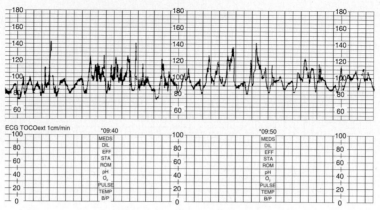

Fig. 4.26 ■ Sinus bradycardia.

beta-blockers for hypertension, which is contraindicated in pregnancy.

Tachycardia

Tachycardia with a baseline rate greater than 160 bpm should prompt a search for other suspicious features such as absence of accelerations, poor baseline variability and decelerations. Tachycardia is not uncommon in pre-term fetuses owing to the earlier maturation of the sympathetic nervous system. With increasing maturity of the fetus the baseline heart rate gradually falls and at term is often between 110 and 140 bpm. Fetal tachycardia may be due to fetal movement or increased sympathetic tone caused by arousal associated with noise, pain or acoustic stimulation. Fetal hypoxia, hypovolaemia and anaemia are pathological causes of tachycardia. Maternal sympathomimetic activation due to pain or anxiety may lead to fetal tachycardia, as can dehydration leading to poor uterine perfusion. Pain relief, reassurance and hydration may be expected to reverse this. Administration of betamimetic drugs to inhibit pre-term labour increases sympathetic activity, whereas anti-cholinergic drugs such as atropine abolish parasympathetic activity through the vagal nerve, resulting in tachycardia.

FALSE OR ERRONEOUS BASELINE BECAUSE OF DOUBLE COUNTING OF LOW BASELINE FHR

In normal circumstances, the atrium and ventricle beat almost simultaneously, followed by the next complete cardiac movement of the atrium and ventricle. The reflected ultrasound from these two chambers, or even from one of the walls (atrium, ventricle or the valves), is used by the machine to compute the FHR. When the FHR is slow, at 70–80 bpm, there is a longer time interval between the atrial and the ventricular contractions. The machine recognizes each of the reflected sounds (one from the ventricle and the other from the atrium) as two separate beats and computes the rate, which may mimic the FHR, as it will be in the expected range for a normal fetal heart. For most observers the sound generated will also give an impression that the FHR is within the normal range; this is because the heart sounds from the machine are always the same for every baby – they are electronic noise. During the false counting or 'doubling' of the FHR episode, listening with a fetal stethoscope will reveal the true situation. The suspicion that something is amiss will be aroused by the FHR tracing, which may show a steady baseline of 140 bpm but at times will be 70 bpm. Because it is a double-counting phenomenon the upper rate on the recording paper will be exactly double that of the lower rate and can be easily checked by auscultation. Such a trace can also be due to the machine recognizing an atrial rate of 140 bpm and a ventricular rate of 70 bpm at different times in a case with complete heart block (Fig. 4.27). The mother may have an autoimmune disorder. Doubling the rate is a phenomenon dependent on the use of ultrasound monitoring. A fetal electrode will not show this effect and should therefore be used if in doubt. A situation of bradycardia with the doubling effect may be observed in a sick fetus as an acute episode and a pre-terminal event.

Beware of double counting.

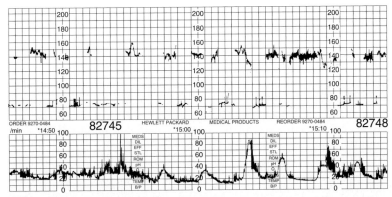

Fig. 4.27 ■ Intermittent double counting – heart block in maternal systemic lupus erythematosus.

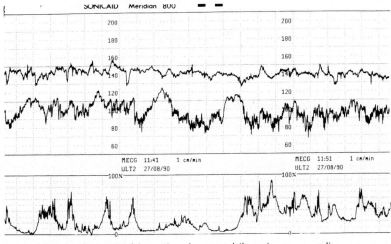

Fig. 4.28 ■ Fetal (upper) and maternal (lower) trace recording.

Bradycardia: Fetal or Maternal?

A record of the maternal heart rate made by using the external ECG mode of the monitor by applying maternal skin electrodes, supplied with the equipment, is shown in Figure 4.28. This is identical to fetal recordings (see Fig. 4.28, upper trace), and mimics FHR when there is maternal anxiety or with betamimetic therapy for pre-term labour, which results in a maternal tachycardia. With current fetal monitors that have facilities for maternal pulse oximetry, the maternal heart rate can be recorded, and better still if 'smart pulse' facility with the external transducer is available (see Fig. 2.8). If the woman reports with reduced fetal movements she may have a tachycardia due to anxiety, and this may be mistaken for the actual FHR while the fetus

is dead. Note that the lower trace, which is maternal, accelerates and has variability, as does the fetal trace.

If you do not have a modern monitor that displays a reliable maternal as well as a fetal pulse then always use the fetal stethoscope before applying the machine. This is the advice of the Medical Devices Agency of the UK.

When the fetus is dead the ultrasound may be inadvertently directed at maternal vessels. The technical quality of this trace is usually poor with incomplete continuity. In such circumstances, it is prudent to verify the presence of the fetal heart activity by auscultation, confirming it with an ultrasound scan if there is doubt.

If two baseline rates appear that do not show the 'doubling' phenomenon the transducer may be picking up the fetal heart at one time and the maternal pulse

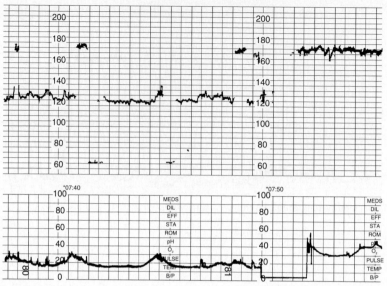

Fig. 4.29 ■ Maternal (120 bpm) and fetal (170 bpm) tachycardia – ultrasound mode.

at another time. The trace in Figure 4.29 was recorded in pre-term labour treated with betamimetic drugs showing fetal and maternal tachycardia. This should be verified by counting the maternal pulse at the wrist and by auscultating the fetal heart simultaneously. The findings should be documented on the CTG paper for clinical and medico-legal purposes.

Fetal Arrhythmia

Complete fetal heart block may be recorded as a stable bradycardia and may give a trace as shown in Figure 4.27. Incomplete heart block is more of a dilemma. Both diagnoses should be substantiated by a detailed B-mode ultrasound scan and further investigation. A heart block must be a proportion of the actual rate (2:1, 3:1) and this should be analysed. Confirmed heart block should prompt a search in the mother's blood for autoimmune antibodies even if she is asymptomatic. Fetal heart block compromises intrapartum surveillance and alternative methods to electronic fetal monitoring should be used (e.g., clinical sense, fetal blood sampling, Doppler blood-flow study).

Occasional dropped beats or ectopic beats are a relatively common phenomenon in normal fetuses; however, more persistent arrhythmias can be associated with hypoxia.

PROBLEMS ASSOCIATED WITH INTERPRETATION OF TRACES

In the past much time and effort has been spent on categorizing decelerations into 'early', 'late' and 'variable', rather than interpreting the trace as a whole in relation to the clinical situation. A given trace may be acceptable as normal in the late first stage but not in the early first stage of labour. At times it is difficult to classify the decelerations as early, variable or late. Often they may have mixed features of variable and late decelerations. It is far more important to categorize any trace as normal, suspicious or pathological. The FIGO[1] and NICE[2] recommendations for the classification of the features of the CTG and the CTG as a whole are described in Chapter 6.

Figure 4.30 shows a trace with tachycardia, no accelerations, reduced baseline variability and repetitive decelerations. Clinically the fetus is post-term and the mother is in early labour. This is a grossly abnormal trace demanding intervention. The decelerations may be analysed as variable because of the precipitous fall in the baseline rate characteristic of cord compression and because the decelerations vary in shape and size. They may be considered to be late because of the lateness in recovery. However, even when the decelerations

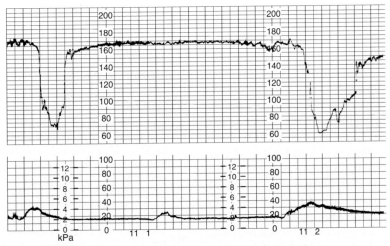

Fig. 4.30 ■ Grossly abnormal features – pathological trace.

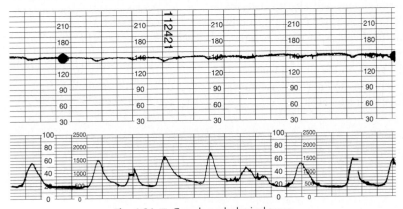

Fig. 4.31 ■ Grossly pathological trace.

are ignored the trace is abnormal because there are no accelerations, the baseline rate is greater than 160 bpm and the baseline variability is less than 5 bpm. There should be no hesitation in classifying this trace as pathological. Those who have limited knowledge of the pathophysiology of FHR may spend time arguing about the nature of the decelerations without concentrating on the whole trace and the clinical picture.

Intervention is mandatory.

Figure 4.31 shows a pathological trace, but this is difficult to recognize unless one is aware of the exception to the rule of interpreting FHR traces. The rate can be within the normal range (110–160 bpm) but with reduced baseline variability (<<5 bpm) and repeated

late decelerations less than 15 bpm. This is an ominous picture unless the trace has shown recent reactive segments. The clinical picture has to be considered and, at times, an immediate delivery is opted for on clinical grounds. All the features of a given trace must be considered before it is categorized as normal, suspicious/non-reassuring or pathological/abnormal. The subsequent management of patients depends on this.

Shallow decelerations with reduced baseline variability in the 'quiet epoch' following an 'active epoch' with accelerations have been found to be associated with fetal breathing episodes.[5] If, on admission or commencement of the CTG, there is reduced baseline variability and shallow decelerations, one should look for clinical symptoms and signs that might suggest possible hypoxia or other insults (e.g., reduced or absent fetal movements, infection, intrauterine growth restriction, prolonged pregnancy or vaginal bleeding). If no such symptoms or signs are evident but mother is at, or close to, term and is in early labour, an artificial rupture of membranes may reveal thick meconium with scanty fluid highlighting possible compromise and the need for delivery. In the absence of the above and if the baseline variability is at least 3–5 bpm, it may be acceptable to wait for up to 40 min and a maximum of 90 min for the next active epoch with accelerations to become evident. In early labour, if facilities permit, use of ultrasound to observe the quantity of amniotic fluid, fetal body or breathing movements and fetal tone may be useful. If it is in the antenatal period and the fetus is pre-term, it may be prudent to undertake the above biophysical assessment and also to determine fetal growth and examine the blood flow in the umbilical arteries and the fetal vessels. If these facilities or expertise are not available then consideration should be given to delivery based on the clinical features and fetal maturity. Accelerations and normal baseline variability are the hallmarks of fetal health.

- A hypoxic fetus can have a normal baseline rate, other features being abnormal.
- In the absence of accelerations, repeated shallow decelerations (below 15 bpm) are ominous when baseline variability is less than 5 bpm.

REFERENCES

[1] Ayres-de-Campos D, Arulkumaran S, FIGO Intrapartum Fetal Monitoring Expert Consensus Panel. FIGO consensus guidelines on intrapartum fetal monitoring: physiology of fetal oxygenation and the main goals of intrapartum fetal monitoring. Int J Gynecol Obstet 2015;131:5–8.

[2] National Institute for Health and Care Excellence (NICE). Intrapartum care for healthy mothers and babies - Fetal monitoring. Available: https://www.nice.org.uk/guidance/indevelopment/gid-ng10174. [accessed 25.11.2022].

[3] Wheeler T, Murills A. Patterns of fetal heart rate during normal pregnancy. Br J Obstet Gynaecol 1978;85:18–27.

[4] Spencer JAD, Johnson P. Fetal heart rate variability changes and fetal behavioural cycles during labour. Br J Obstet Gynaecol 1986;93:314–321.

[5] Schifrin B, Artenos J, Lyseight N. Late-onset fetal cardiac decelerations associated with fetal breathing movements. J Matern Fetal Neonatal Med 2002;12(4):253–259.

5

PATHOPHYSIOLOGY OF FETAL HEART RATE (FHR) PATTERNS

DONALD GIBB ■ SABARATNAM ARULKUMARAN

Control of the fetal heart rate (FHR) and the associated features of accelerations, decelerations and baseline variability is complex (Fig. 5.1). The baseline FHR is determined by the spontaneous activity of the pacemaker in the sinoatrial (SA) node in the atrium. This specialized area of the myocardium initiates the fastest rate and determines the 'baseline' rate in the normal heart. The atrioventricular (AV) node situated on the AV septum has a slower rate of activity and generates the idioventricular rhythm seen in complete heart block. Under the circumstances of complete heart block, the ventricle beats at 60–80 beats per minute (bpm).

The FHR is modulated by a number of stimuli. Central nervous system influence is important with cortical and subcortical influences not under voluntary control. We cannot alter our heart rate at will. The cardioregulatory centre in the brain stem also plays a part. Other physiological factors regulate the heart rate, such as circulatory catecholamines, chemoreceptors, baroreceptors and their interplay with the autonomic nervous system.[1]

The efferent component of the autonomic nervous system is composed of the sympathetic and parasympathetic systems. There is a constant input from these systems varying from millisecond to millisecond. Sympathetic impulses drive the heart rate to increase, while parasympathetic impulses have the opposite effect. If we are confronted with a frightening situation our heart rate involuntarily increases. This puts us under stress, sometimes distress; however, it is an adaptive mechanism preparing us for fight or flight – the sympathetic response. On the contrary, if we are

feeling very relaxed and happy at home in the evening after a busy day then our heart rate will decrease on account of parasympathetic stimulation.

Electronic FHR monitors compute the heart rate based on averaged intervals between beats extrapolated to what the rate would be if that beat interval remained constant. The machine produces a rate recording after being applied for only a few seconds. However, autonomic impulses immediately and constantly take effect, changing the beat intervals and immediately altering the heart rate. This is how baseline variability is generated and it indicates integrity of the autonomic nervous system (Fig. 5.2). Baseline variability is actually seen on the tracing. If it is greatly magnified, individual beats and beat-to-beat variation can be seen with special equipment used for physiological studies (Fig. 5.3). In practice though, baseline variability is the preferred term. The sympathetic nervous system and the parasympathetic or vagal system have the specific effect of generating baseline variability. Suppression of vagal impulses by a drug such as atropine causes tachycardia and reduces baseline variability. Physiological mechanisms are complex and incompletely understood. The autonomic nervous system is sensitive to hypoxia at a critical level for the fetus and changes in this response are therefore used as important indicators of well-being. The sympathetic and parasympathetic systems mature at slightly different rates with respect to gestational age. The sympathetic system matures faster and this results in marginally faster baseline rates in the pre-term period. It is of some interest that male fetuses have slightly faster heart rates than female fetuses; however, this is of absolutely no diagnostic

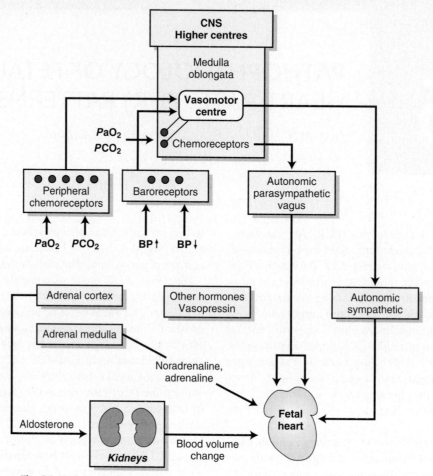

Fig. 5.1 ■ Control of the fetal heart. *CNS,* central nervous system; *BP,* blood pressure.

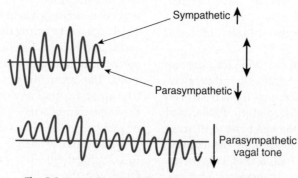

Fig. 5.2 ■ Baseline variability – autonomic modulation.

value or clinical significance. Before 34 weeks' gestation a higher baseline rate is to be expected. Normal baseline variability suggests good autonomic control and therefore little likelihood of hypoxia.

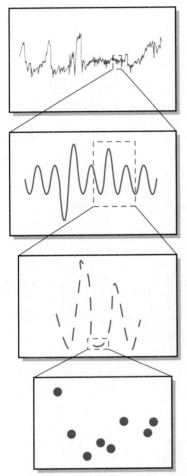

Fig. 5.3 ▪ Baseline variability – beat-to-beat variation.

PATHOPHYSIOLOGICAL MECHANISMS OF DECELERATIONS

An understanding of the maintenance of autonomic control and the mechanisms of decelerations is important. The following illustrations show the effects of contractions on the fetus and blood flow in diagrammatic form (Figs 5.4–5.9).

Early decelerations are early in timing with respect to the uterine contractions and this is therefore a better term than type 1 dips. They are most commonly due to compression of the fetal head. A rise in intracranial pressure is associated with stimulation of the vagal nerve and bradycardia. This may be caused by a uterine contraction and the sequence of events in this situation is shown in Figures 5.5–5.9. Head compression decelerations are most frequently seen in the late stages of labour when descent of the head is occurring. Indeed, on some occasions the onset of the second stage of labour can be deduced from the tracing. Decelerations due to head compression are seen at the time of vaginal examination and also when artificial rupture of the membranes has been performed. Early decelerations with contractions are symmetrical and bell-shaped (Fig. 5.10). The clinical situation should be reviewed to ensure that head compression is a likely explanation at that time. If not, and if the trace is atypical, then an apparently innocuous early deceleration may be an atypical variable deceleration and may be pathological. In one case, the obstetric registrar reported that a young West Indian nullipara suffering from sickle cell disease at term but with abdominal size and scan suggesting intrauterine growth restriction was 'niggling' but not yet in established labour. The fetal head was unengaged. He reported the trace (Fig. 5.11) as

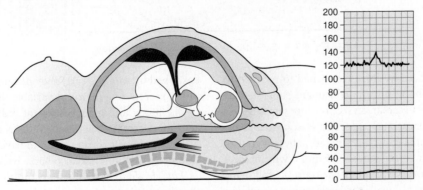

Fig. 5.4 ▪ Diagrammatic representation of fetus, placenta and blood flow.

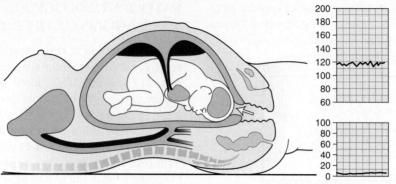

Fig. 5.5 ■ Early deceleration – start of contraction.

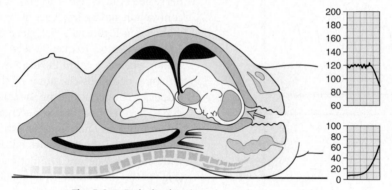

Fig. 5.6 ■ Early deceleration – increasing contraction.

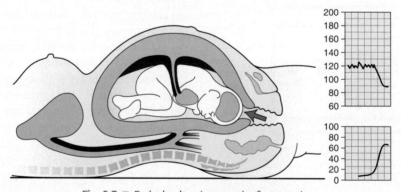

Fig. 5.7 ■ Early deceleration – peak of contraction.

showing early decelerations. He wished to proceed to induction of labour, but the consultant suggested he proceed directly to caesarean section. The registrar was surprised but learned an important lesson on delivering a significantly growth-restricted baby covered in meconium with Apgar scores of 5 and 6 who made a satisfactory recovery. Review of the trace the following day showed that although the decelerations might be described by some as early they do show late recovery of the second one (atypical variable deceleration), no accelerations and a suggestion of reduced variability after the second deceleration. What is more important is that this fetus had no reason to have head compression in early labour and also had a background of risk.

Late decelerations are late in timing with respect to the uterine contraction and are therefore best described

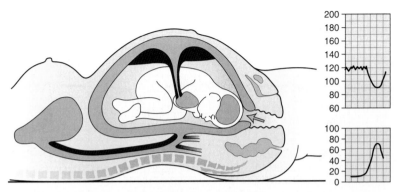

Fig. 5.8 ▪ Early deceleration – decreasing contraction.

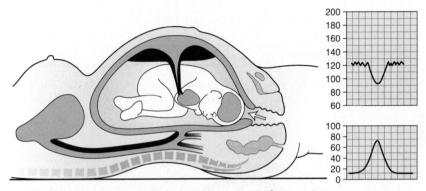

Fig. 5.9 ▪ Early deceleration – end of contraction.

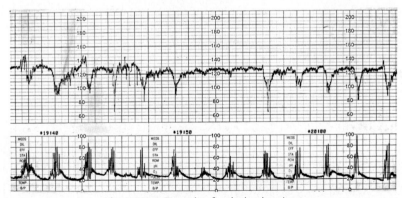

Fig. 5.10 ▪ Example of early decelerations.

as such rather than as type 2 dips. The suggested patho-physiological mechanism of such decelerations is shown in Figures 5.12–5.14. There is a reservoir of oxygenated blood in the retroplacental space. The size of this space varies and is smaller in intrauterine growth restriction. Poor blood flow to the uteroplacental space is character-istic of fetuses with intrauterine growth restriction. As

a contraction begins the fetus uses up the reservoir of oxygen in the retroplacental space. Due to the restricted supply of blood a hypoxic deceleration begins (usually 20 seconds (s) after the onset of the contraction), it con-tinues through the contraction and it does not recover fully until sometime after the contraction when full oxy-genation has been restored. The speed of recovery on

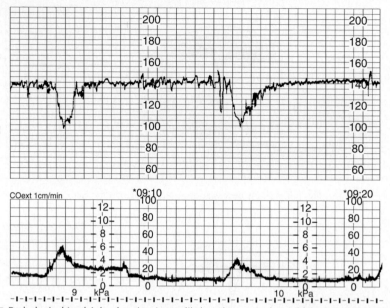

Fig. 5.11 ■ Pathological 'early' deceleration (more likely to be atypical variable) – head 4/5 to 5/5 palpable.

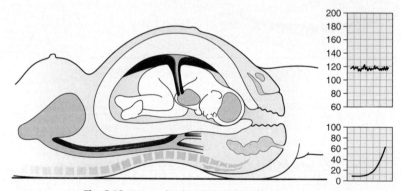

Fig. 5.12 ■ Late deceleration – start of contraction.

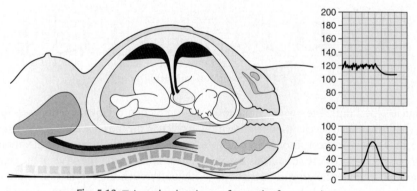

Fig. 5.13 ■ Late deceleration – after peak of contraction.

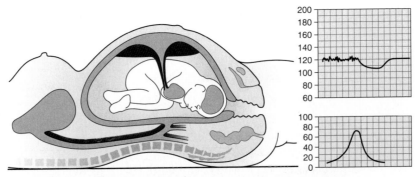

Fig. 5.14 ■ Late deceleration – end of contraction.

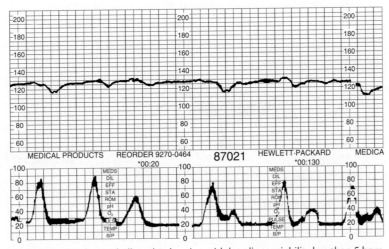

Fig. 5.15 ■ Ominous shallow deceleration with baseline variability less than 5 bpm.

the ascending limb may reflect the blood flow and the resilience of the fetus. In a non-hypoxic fetus there is increased variability during a deceleration on account of autonomic response. When hypoxia develops there is a tendency to reduced variability.

BASELINE VARIABILITY AND DECELERATIONS – EXCEPTION TO THE RULE

A deceleration is defined when the FHR decelerates by more than 15 beats from the baseline for more than 15 s. However, this rule does not apply when the baseline variability is less than 5 beats and any deceleration even less than 15 beats from the baseline could be ominous (Fig. 5.15) unless otherwise proven in a non-reactive trace.

Variable decelerations are the most common type of deceleration and are called variable because they vary in shape, size and sometimes in timing with respect to each other. They vary because they are a manifestation of compression of the umbilical cord and it is compressed in a slightly different way each time. On some occasions it may not be compressed at all and there is no deceleration with that particular contraction. Variable decelerations are more often seen when the amniotic fluid volume is reduced. In North America, they are referred to as cord compression decelerations.

The mechanism is illustrated in Figures 5.16–5.20. The umbilical vein has a thinner wall and lower intraluminal pressure than the umbilical arteries (see Fig. 5.16). When compression occurs the blood flow through the vein is interrupted before that through the artery. The fetus therefore loses some of its

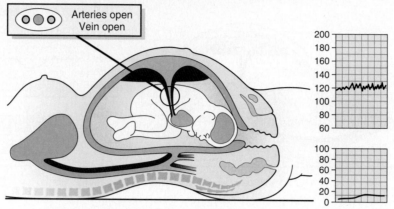

Fig. 5.16 ■ Umbilical cord, fetus and placenta – normal circulation.

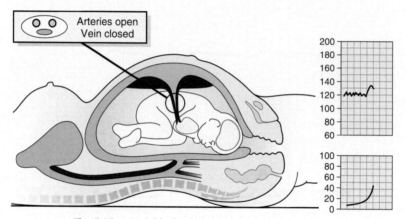

Fig. 5.17 ■ Variable deceleration – start of contraction.

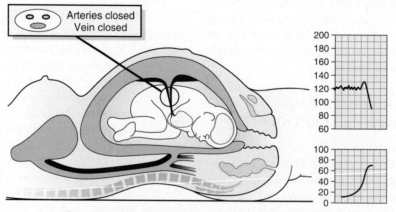

Fig. 5.18 ■ Variable deceleration – increasing contraction.

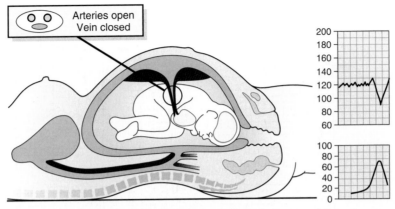

Fig. 5.19 ▪ Variable deceleration – decreasing contraction.

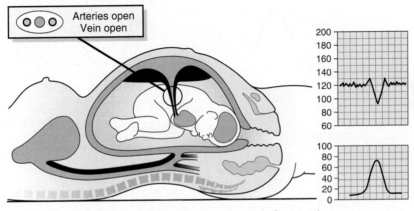

Fig. 5.20 ▪ Variable deceleration – end of contraction.

circulating blood volume. When a healthy individual or fetus loses some of its circulating blood volume the natural response effected by the autonomic nervous system is a rise in pulse rate to compensate. A small rise in the FHR therefore appears at the start of a variable deceleration when the umbilical artery is not compromised (see Fig. 5.17). After that the umbilical arteries are also occluded, the circulation is relatively restored, followed by an increase in systemic pressure, the baroreceptors are stimulated and there is a precipitous fall in the FHR (see Fig. 5.18). The deceleration is at its nadir with both vessels occluded. During release of the cord compression, arterial flow is restored first with a consequent autonomically mediated sharp rise in heart rate (see Fig. 5.19) due to systemic hypotension of blood being pumped out culminating in a small rise in FHR after

the deceleration (see Fig. 5.20). These rises in FHR before and after decelerations are called shouldering. Whatever they are called, they are a manifestation of a fetus coping well with cord compression. The way the cord is being compressed will vary depending exactly on how it is positioned with respect to the structure compressing it. On the same basis, variable decelerations may change if the posture of the mother is changed. Normal well-grown fetuses can tolerate cord compression for a considerable length of time before they become hypoxic. Small growth-restricted fetuses do not have the same resilience.

1. To assess this process it is necessary to analyse the features of the decelerations and also the character of the trace as it evolves. Figure 5.21 shows normal shouldering.

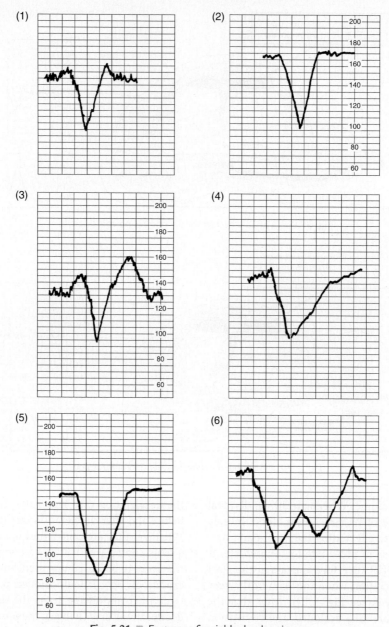

Fig. 5.21 ■ Features of variable decelerations.

2. Exaggeration of shouldering or overshoot (indicates that additional circulations are needed to normalize) – which is thought to be prepathological.
3. Loss of shouldering – pathological.
4. Smoothing of the baseline variability within the deceleration – which is associated with loss of variability at the baseline and is therefore pathological.

5. Late recovery (variable and late deceleration components merged together) – which has the same pathological significance as late deceleration.
6. Biphasic deceleration (variable and late decelerations seen as separate components) – requiring the same consideration as a late deceleration.

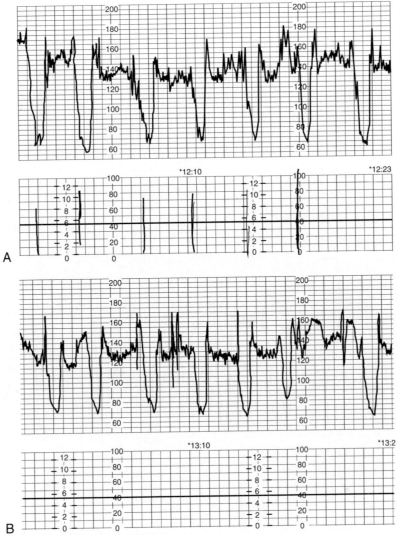

Fig. 5.22 ■ Two CTGs recorded 60 min apart, showing variable decelerations. There is no rise in the baseline rate or variability. Occasional decelerations with beat loss greater than 60 and duration greater than 60 s need close observation.

7. If the duration of the deceleration is more than 60 s and the depth is greater than 60 beats, progressive hypoxia becomes more likely.

At times a fetus may have more than one stress operating (e.g., a fetus with intrauterine growth restriction may have cord compression due to oligohydramnios and late decelerations due to reduced amount of retroplacental blood behind the small and partially infarcted placenta). The most critical feature, however,

is the evolution of the trace with time. A change in the baseline rate and change in the baseline variability are the key signs of developing hypoxia and acidosis.

Figure 5.22 shows two strips of cardiotocograph (CTG) 60 minutes (min) apart. In spite of marked variable decelerations, the baseline rate and baseline variability are maintained. So long as adequate progress is being made toward delivery this trace need not cause concern. Figure 5.23 also shows two strips of trace 20 min apart but with quite different features.

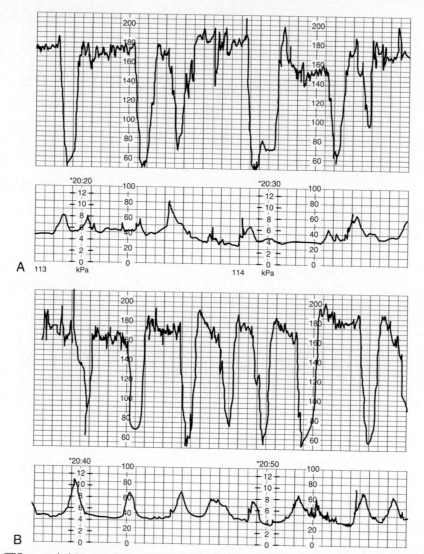

Fig. 5.23 ■ Two CTGs recorded 20 min apart: (A) variable decelerations with abnormal features (duration >60 s, depth >60 beats; tachycardia) (abnormal trace); (B) suggestive of distress (tachycardia and reduced baseline variability).

The progression to a tachycardia with reduced variability suggests developing hypoxia. The time required for a fetus with a previously normal trace to become acidotic related to different patterns of the FHR has been studied.[2] In many cases, it may take over 100 min. Medical staff should have time enough to identify the problem and act effectively.

At times, it may be difficult to decide whether the decelerations are early, late or variable. It is not only the deceleration itself that is critical but also the evolution of the trace with time and the clinical features. The baseline rate between decelerations, the baseline variability and the presence or absence of accelerations are all critical.

CLASSIFICATION OF FETAL HEART RATE PATTERN

The National Institute for Health and Care Excellence (NICE) and International Federation of Obstetrics and

Gynaecology (FIGO) guidelines recommend classifying the individual features of baseline rate, baseline variability, decelerations and accelerations as reassuring, non-reassuring or abnormal (see Ch. 6). The whole CTG trace is then classified as normal or reassuring, non-reassuring or suspicious, and abnormal or pathological. A summary of the above is given in Box 5.1.

A sinusoidal pattern is a regular heart rate with cyclic changes in the FHR baseline like a sine wave, the characteristics of the pattern being that the frequency is less than 6 cycles per min, the amplitude is at least 10 bpm and the duration should be 10 min or longer. Additional details are given in Chapter 6.

A *normal* classification of the trace implies that the trace assures fetal health. *Suspicious* indicates that continued observation or additional simple tests are required to ensure fetal health. *Pathological* warrants some action in the form of additional tests or delivery depending on the clinical picture. If one of the features of the CTG is abnormal, possible remedial action should be taken and, at times, a short period of observation of the trace may be appropriate if there are no clinical risk factors like intrauterine growth restriction, meconium or infection. If there are clinical risk factors or two abnormal features, additional testing such as fetal scalp blood sampling to elucidate the fetal condition, or delivery, may be more prudent if remedial action does not correct the abnormal features of the trace. If three features of the CTG are abnormal, one should consider delivery unless spontaneous delivery is imminent, or perform fetal scalp blood sampling to elucidate the fetal condition. The degree of abnormality of the CTG, clinical risk factors, parity, current cervical dilatation and the rate of progress of labour should determine the decisions to observe, perform a fetal scalp blood sample or deliver promptly. Table 6.1 describes the recommended actions with different categories of FHR patterns observed.

The expression *fetal distress* should be reconsidered. A trace that is not normal may result from physiological, iatrogenic or pathological causes. The clinical situation and the dynamic evolution of features of the trace with time will clarify the situation.

The underlying principle is to detect fetal compromise using the concept of 'fetal distress' very critically. In all situations, it is consideration of the overall clinical picture that will provide the clues as to whether true fetal compromise is present. Many suspicious CTGs are generated by healthy fetuses demonstrating the ability to respond to stress. For the purposes of clinical decision-making, so far, scoring systems or computer analysis have not been found to be useful, particularly in the intrapartum period. Results of a large randomized control trial consisting of 45,000 women (INFANT study) has shown that computer-assisted interpretation of CTG did not result in better neonatal outcome or reduction in emergency caesarean section. There are several research groups working on 'machine learning' (ML) using the clinical and the CTG information to see whether current practice can be improved by ML to reduce caesarean sections and babies born with poor outcome.

PRACTICAL HINTS TO IDENTIFY GRADUAL DETERIORATION OF FETAL CONDITION (FIG. 5.24)

With gradual deterioration of the fetal condition, one observes gradual rise in the baseline rate and reduction of baseline variability, that is with progressive hypoxia which is seen in the trace below. If one draws a vertical line at the onset and offset of the contractions and the deceleration with sudden decline and back to normal baseline rate falls within these two lines, then it is a typical variable deceleration. This is seen with the first contraction on the CTG below. With increasing hypoxia, the FHR returns to the baseline rate much later than the vertical line drawn from the offset of the contraction – that is atypical variable deceleration as seen with the second contraction on the CTG trace below. With increasing hypoxia there is an increase in depth and duration of the deceleration as observed

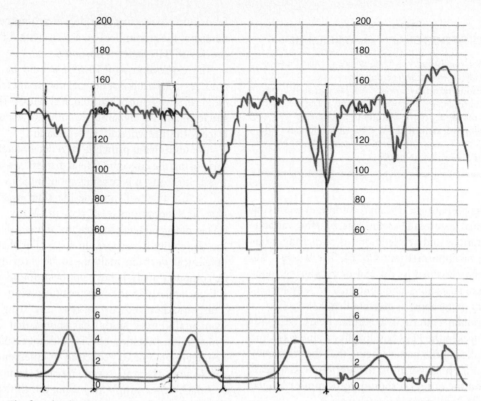

Fig. 5.24 ■ The first deceleration is within the onset and offset of the contraction. Gradually decelerations become deeper and wider with reduction of inter-decelleration interval along with rise in baseline rate and reduction in baseline variability.

with the decelerations with the subsequent contractions. As a result of increasing duration of decelerations, the inter-deceleration intervals when the FHR returns to its normal rate are gradually reduced resulting in increasingly poor perfusion in the fetal circulation. This causes hypoxia resulting in catecholamine surge resulting in gradual increase in baseline rate. The FIGO or NICE CTG guidelines provide information on basic interpretation. Consideration of physiological evolution of the FHR should help us better decide on the need for intervention and when. A pathological FHR does not become better with progress of time but gets worse unless there was an offending factor like an oxytocin infusion causing too many contractions. This can be stopped to allow the heart rate to recover.

The first deceleration is within the vertical lines from the onset and offset of the contraction. Gradually decelerations become deeper and wider with reduction

of inter-deceleration interval along with rise in baseline rate and reduction in baseline variability – signs of increasing hypoxia (see Fig. 5.24).

PRACTICAL HINTS TO IDENTIFY POSSIBLE ACUTE DETERIORATION OF FETAL CONDITION (FIG. 5.25)

When there is a prolonged period of cord compression with each contraction (as in cord prolapse or loops of cord tightly round the neck in the second stage with descent of head) the decelerations are prolonged equal to or greater than 90 to 120 s with less than half that period at the baseline rate resulting in less perfusion to the fetus as seen in Figure 5.25. In such a situation, acute deterioration of the fetal condition would be reflected by the gradual decline of the baseline FHR that does not return to the earlier baseline rate but to

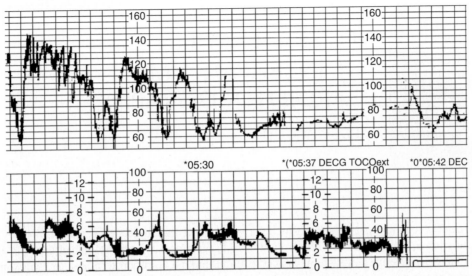

Fig. 5.25 ■ Decelerations are prolonged (>90 s) with brief recovery to baseline rate (<30 s) and after each deceleration the baseline rate is becoming significantly less suggesting acute deterioration of fetal condition.

significantly lower FHR following subsequent decelerations – as seen above. With time this progressive drop in the FHR may lead to bradycardia and asystole with the baby born with Apgar score of 0 at 1 and 5 min. With such an occurrence if the CTG or Doppler shows a recovery to a higher rate this could be maternal heart rate as a 'worsening pattern suddenly does not become better'. It is a dilemma in the second stage when the FHR shows prolonged decelerations with less than half to third time of the duration of deceleration spent at the baseline rate whilst the head is progressively descending and spontaneous vaginal delivery is anticipated. If the baseline is not returning to its original baseline rate and the FHR in between decelerations is gradually declining, assisted birth may be prudent unless vaginal delivery is imminent.

REFERENCES

[1] Parer JT. In defense of FHR monitoring's specificity. Cont Obstet Gynaecol 1982;19:228–234.

[2] Fleischer A, Shulman H, Jagani N, et al. The development of fetal acidosis in the presence of an abnormal fetal heart rate tracing. I. The average for gestation age fetus. Am J Obstet Gynecol 1982;144:55–60.

[3] The INFANT Collaborative Group. Computerised interpretation of fetal heart rate during labour (INFANT): a randomised controlled trial. Lancet 2017;389:1719–1729.

6

INTERPRETATION OF INTRAPARTUM CARDIOTOCOGRAPHY

DIOGO AYRES DE CAMPOS

Labour is a rapidly evolving process, during which the frequency, duration and strength of uterine contractions usually increases. Uterine contractions can cause varying degrees of compression of intrauterine vessels and of the umbilical cord, with the resulting reduction in fetal oxygenation. These can be temporary and reversible events, or a slowly/rapidly progressing phenomenon.

Cardiotocography (CTG), from the Greek words *kardia* meaning heart, and *tokos* meaning labour/childbirth, is the term that best describes the continuous monitoring of fetal heart rate (FHR) and uterine contraction signals. The basic principles of the technology were developed more than 50 years ago, primarily to identify signs of reduced fetal oxygenation during labour, thereby allowing the use of appropriate obstetric interventions to avoid adverse outcomes, such as perinatal death, hypoxic-ischaemic encephalopathy and long-term sequelae such as cerebral palsy.

By correctly interpreting CTG tracings, healthcare professionals can clearly identify fetuses that are being adequately oxygenated during labour. With less certainty, they can identify those that are being exposed to mechanical stress but remain compensated, and those that have exhausted their compensatory mechanisms and are undergoing intrapartum hypoxia.

The International Federation of Obstetrics and Gynecology (FIGO) guidelines on intrapartum fetal monitoring represent the widest consensus ever reached in this field. In addition to reviewing the existing evidence on intrapartum fetal monitoring, the authors made efforts to use an accessible language and

to make the guidelines as simple, objective and easy to remember as possible. One of the main aims was to promote a common terminology that would be useful for research and for improvement of clinical care throughout the world. By including management options in the classification table, the ultimate goal was to contribute to a reduction in perinatal mortality and long-term sequelae, while at the same time avoiding unnecessary obstetrical intervention. The latter was another major aim of the guidelines, and a large emphasis was given to the definition of reversible versus irreversible causes of fetal hypoxia and to the adoption of measures that improve fetal oxygenation (i.e., reducing or stopping oxytocin perfusion, administration of acute tocolysis agents, changing maternal position, correction of maternal hypotension) before undertaking obstetric interventions (i.e., operative vaginal birth or caesarean section).

For adequate CTG interpretation and subsequent clinical decision, in addition to CTG analysis and classification, healthcare professionals need to take into account the overall clinical picture. This includes evaluating the rate of labour progress, individual characteristics of the fetus (i.e., fetal growth restriction, oligohydramnios), as well as maternal conditions (i.e., pre-eclampsia, vaginal bleeding, pyrexia, etc.). It is important to remember that fetal neurological damage is not just caused by hypoxia. Fetal systemic inflammation, as occurs with clinical chorioamnionitis, has a strong correlation with permanent neurological damage, so these aspects also need to be taken into consideration when intervention is considered.

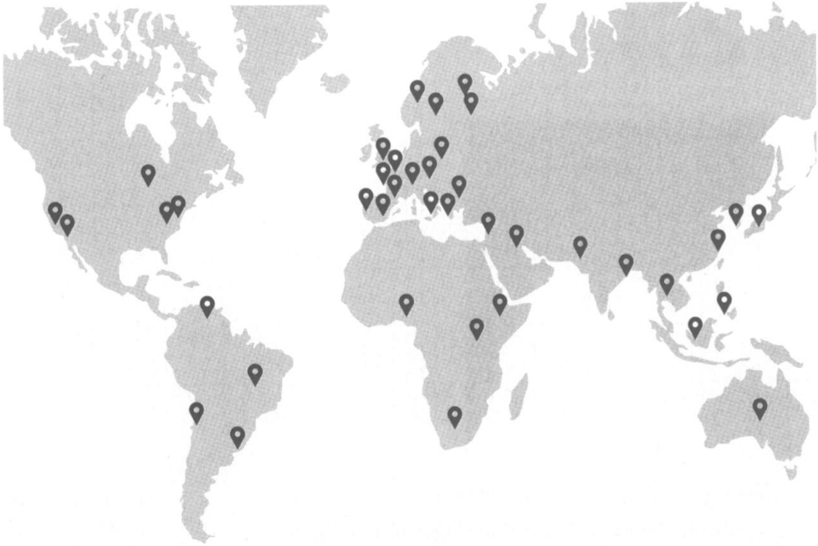

Fig. 6.1 ▪ Geographic representation of the panel members of the 2015 International Federation of Obstetrics and Gynecology consensus guidelines on intrapartum fetal monitoring.

GUIDELINE DEVELOPMENT

The 2015 FIGO consensus guidelines on intrapartum monitoring[1-5] were developed with the purpose of updating the previous FIGO guidelines, published in 1987.[6] The process involved a total of 50 experts, 34 nominated by FIGO national member societies and 16 invited based on their publication record in the field. The process also involved the contribution of chapter authors recommended by the American College of Obstetricians and Gynecologists (ACOG), the Royal College of Obstetricians and Gynaecologists (RCOG), and the International Confederation of Midwives (ICM). A geographical representation of the members of the consensus panel is presented in Figure 6.1.

The consensus process was conducted by email and involved three rounds of agreement for each chapter, followed by a written consent to be included in the panel list. The process involved no internal or external funding and took 10 months to prepare and a further 18 months to conclude. The guidelines have been endorsed by the European Association of Perinatal Medicine (EAPM), the European Board and College of Obstetrics and Gynaecology (EBCOG), the Asia and Oceania Federation of Obstetrics and Gynaecology, the Latin–American Federation of Perinatal Medicine Associations and the Latin–American Federation of Obstetrics and Gynecology Societies, and have been supported by the ACOGs.

In this chapter we provide a brief overview of the concepts presented in the CTG chapter of these guidelines. The full document can be accessed at http://www.ijgo.org/article/S0020-7292(15)00395-1/pdf.

CARDIOTOCOGRAPHY ANALYSIS

CTG analysis starts with an evaluation of basic CTG features followed by overall tracing classification.

Evaluation of Basic Cardiotocography Features

Evaluation of basic CTG features comprises assessment of the FHR baseline, variability, accelerations, decelerations and other patterns, fetal behavioural state and contractions, and this process requires a good comprehension of the underlying physiology.

BASELINE – is the mean level of the most horizontal and less oscillatory FHR segments, estimated in periods of 10 minutes (min; it can vary between different periods) and is expressed in beats per minute (bpm). Care must be taken to identify the fetal behavioural state of active wakefulness (see 'Fetal behavioural states' later), which can lead to an erroneously high baseline estimation (see Fig. 6.8).
Normal baseline – between 110 and 160 bpm.
Tachycardia – baseline greater than 160 bpm for more than 10 min. Maternal pyrexia is the most

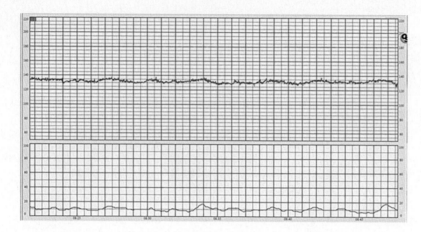

Fig. 6.2 ■ Cardiotocography displaying reduced baseline variability.

frequent cause, but it may also be associated with epidural analgesia, the initial stages of fetal hypoxaemia, administration of beta-agonist drugs, parasympathetic blockers, and fetal arrhythmias such as supraventricular tachycardia and atrial flutter.

Bradycardia – baseline less than 110 bpm for more than 10 min. May be caused by acute fetal hypoxia, maternal hypothermia, administration of beta-blockers and fetal arrhythmias such as atrial–ventricular block.

VARIABILITY – are the oscillations in the FHR signal, evaluated as the average signal bandwidth amplitude in 1-min segments. There is a high degree of subjectivity in visual evaluation of this parameter, and therefore careful re-evaluation is recommended in borderline situations.

Normal variability – between 5 and 25 bpm.

Reduced variability – less than 5 bpm for more than 50 min in baseline segments (Fig. 6.2), or more than 3 min within decelerations. It may be caused by central nervous system hypoxia, previous cerebral injury, infection, administration of central nervous system depressants or parasympathetic blockers. During the fetal behavioural state of deep sleep (see 'Fetal behavioural states' later – Fig. 6.7), variability is usually borderline, and on visual analysis may be classified as reduced. This state seldom exceeds 50 min, so waiting for reversal of the behavioural state will clarify the situation.

Increased variability (**saltatory pattern**) – exceeding 25 bpm for more than 30 min (Fig. 6.3). This pattern has been associated with fetal hypoxia of rapid evolution.

ACCELERATIONS – are abrupt increases in the FHR greater than the baseline, with greater than 15 bpm in amplitude and greater than 15 seconds (s) in duration. Most accelerations coincide with fetal movements and are a sign of a neurologically responsive fetus without hypoxia. Accelerations may have lower amplitude and duration at earlier gestational ages (i.e., before 32 weeks).

DECELERATIONS – are abrupt decreases in the FHR less than the baseline, with greater than 15 bpm in amplitude and greater than 15 s in duration.

Early decelerations – are shallow, short lasting, with normal variability within the deceleration, and coincident with contractions. These are believed to be caused by fetal head compression and do not indicate ongoing fetal hypoxia.

Variable decelerations (**V-shaped**) – have a rapid drop, rapid recovery, good variability within the deceleration and are of varying size, shape and relationship to uterine contractions (Fig. 6.4A). These constitute the majority of decelerations and translate a baroreceptor-mediated response to increased arterial pressure, as occurs with umbilical cord compression. When they have a typical morphology and do not coincide with other FHR changes, they are not associated with important degrees of fetal hypoxia.

Late decelerations (**U-shaped** or with **reduced variability**) – have a gradual onset, or gradual return to the baseline, or have reduced variability

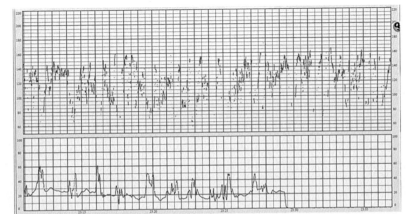

Fig. 6.3 ▪ Cardiotocography displaying increased variability.

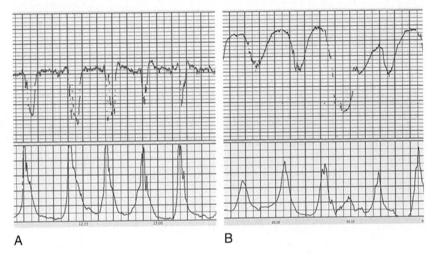

Fig. 6.4 ▪ (A) Cardiotocography (CTG) displaying variable decelerations; (B) CTG displaying late decelerations.

A

B

within the deceleration (Fig. 6.4B); they usually start more than 20 s after the onset of a contraction, have their nadir of the deceleration after the acme of the contraction, and recovery after the end of the contraction. These are indicative of a chemoreceptor-mediated response to sudden fetal hypoxemia. In a tracing with no accelerations and reduced variability, late decelerations should also include those with an amplitude of 10 to 15 bpm.

Prolonged decelerations – are those lasting more than 3 min. These are also likely to include a chemoreceptor-mediated component and thus to indicate sudden fetal hypoxemia. If they exceed 5 min, the FHR is less than 80 bpm and there is reduced variability (Fig. 6.5), they usually indicate acute fetal hypoxia and require urgent intervention.

SINUSOIDAL PATTERN – is a regular, smooth, undulating signal, resembling a sine wave, with an amplitude of 5 to 15 bpm, and a frequency of 3 to 5 cycles per min, lasting more than 30 min (Fig. 6.6A). This pattern occurs more frequently with fetal anaemia but has also been associated with acute fetal hypoxia, infection, cardiac malformations, hydrocephalus and gastroschisis. A similar pattern, but with a more jagged 'saw-tooth' signal, is called **pseudosinusoidal** (Fig. 6.6B). The latter is not associated with hypoxia or other fetal complications but has been described after analgesic administration

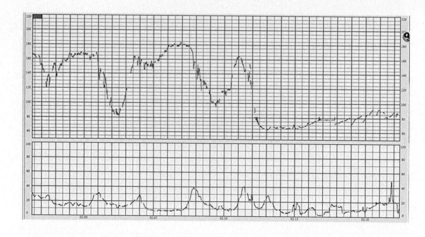

Fig. 6.5 ■ Cardiotocography displaying a prolonged deceleration with more than 5-min duration, requiring urgent intervention.

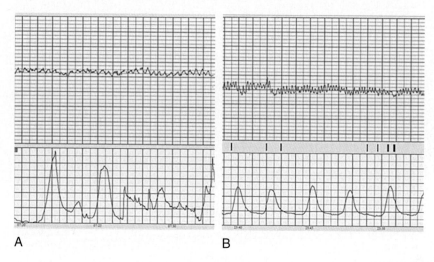

Fig. 6.6 ■ (A) Cardiotocography (CTG) displaying a sinusoidal pattern; (B) a CTG displaying a pseudosinusoidal pattern.

A   B

and during periods of fetal sucking or other mouth movements. It lasts less than 30 min and has normal patterns before and after.

FETAL BEHAVIOURAL STATES – these refer to periods of deep sleep, alternating with active sleep and wakefulness. The occurrence of different behavioural states throughout labour is a hallmark of adequate neurological responsiveness and excludes the occurrence of ongoing hypoxia. Deep sleep can last up to 50 min, and the CTG displays a stable baseline, rare accelerations and borderline variability (Fig. 6.7). Active sleep is the most frequent behavioural state and is represented by frequent accelerations and normal variability. Active wakefulness is rarer and is represented by very frequent accelerations and normal variability (Fig. 6.8). Transitions

between the different patterns become clearer after 32 to 34 weeks of gestation.

CONTRACTIONS – are bell-shaped features, depicting a gradual increase in uterine activity followed by an approximately symmetric decrease, with 45 to 120 s in total duration. With a tocodynamometer, only the frequency of uterine contractions can be reliably evaluated. The presence of more than five contractions in 10 min, in two successive 10-min periods, or averaged over a 30-min period is called tachysystole.

Tracing Classification

Tracings should be classified into one of three classes: normal, suspicious or pathological, according to the criteria presented in Table 6.1. Because of the changing

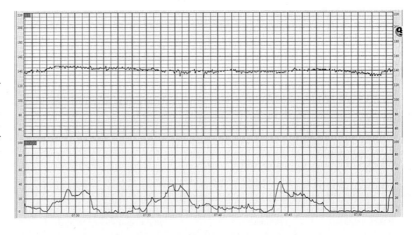

Fig. 6.7 ▪ Cardiotocography representing the fetal behavioural state of deep sleep, which can last up to 50 min. This pattern is difficult to distinguish from that of reduced variability (Fig. 6.2). Only waiting for the end of this state will clarify the situation.

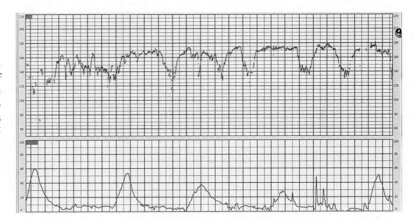

Fig. 6.8 ▪ Cardiotocography representing the fetal behavioural state of active wakefulness. An erroneously high baseline may be identified, if judged to be at the top of accelerations. In this case the baseline is approximately 145 bpm.

nature of CTG signals throughout labour, tracings should be re-evaluated for classification at least once every 30 min.

CLINICAL MANAGEMENT

When tracing characteristics (either basic CTG features or overall CTG classification) are suggestive of an impending or established fetal hypoxia, action is required to avoid an adverse neonatal outcome, but this does not necessarily mean performing an immediate caesarean delivery or instrumental vaginal delivery. When a suspicious or a worsening CTG pattern is identified, the underlying cause for this should be sought, preferably before a pathological tracing develops. If a reversible situation is identified, measures should be taken to correct it and time given for subsequent recovery of fetal oxygenation and the return

of a normal pattern. If the situation does not revert or the CTG pattern continues to deteriorate, the situation needs to be re-evaluated and a rapid delivery decided if a pathological pattern ensues.

Good clinical judgement is required to diagnose the underlying cause of a pathological CTG and to judge the severity and speed of progress of fetal hypoxia. The fetal capacity to withhold the insult, the reversibility of the situation and the probability of recurrence also need to be taken into account. All of these aspects are important for the objective of avoiding an adverse outcome, balanced against the risks of unnecessary obstetric intervention. When there is doubt about the occurrence of fetal hypoxia, adjunctive technologies may be used to clarify the situation further, and these are considered in a separate chapter of the guidelines, which can be accessed at www.ijgo.org/article/S0020-7292(15)00396-3.pdf.

TABLE 6.1

Cardiotocography Classification Criteria, Interpretation and Recommended Management[a]

	Normal	Suspicious	Pathological
Baseline	110–160 bpm	Lacking at least one characteristic of normality, but with no pathological features	<100 bpm
Variability	5–25 bpm		Reduced variability Increased variability Sinusoidal pattern
Decelerations	No repetitive[b] decelerations		Repetitive[b] late or prolonged decelerations for >30 min (or >20 min if reduced variability). Deceleration >5 min
Interpretation	No hypoxia	Low probability of hypoxia	High probability of hypoxia
Clinical management	No intervention necessary to improve fetal oxygenation state	Action to correct reversible causes if identified, close monitoring or adjunctive methods	Immediate action to correct reversible causes, adjunctive methods, or if this is not possible expedite delivery In acute situations, immediate delivery should be accomplished

[a]The absence of accelerations during labour is of uncertain significance.
[b]Decelerations are repetitive in nature when they are associated with more than 50% of uterine contractions.

Reversible Causes of Fetal Hypoxia

Excessive uterine activity: is the most frequent cause of FHR abnormalities and can be detected by identifying tachysystole on the CTG tracing or by palpating the uterine fundus. It is usually reversed by reducing or stopping oxytocin infusion, and/or by starting acute tocolysis. During the second stage of labour, maternal pushing can also contribute to decreased placental perfusion, so the mother should be asked to stop pushing until the situation is reversed.

Aortocaval compression: caused by the pregnant uterus, is frequent in the supine position and may result in reduced placental perfusion. Changing the maternal position, by asking her to turn onto her side, sit up or stand up, is frequently followed by normalization of the CTG pattern.

Sudden maternal hypotension: most frequently occurs after epidural or spinal analgesia and is usually reversible by rapid fluid administration and/or an intravenous ephedrine bolus.

Maternal respiratory or circulatory complications: some of these situations may be reversible in nature (e.g., severe asthma, haemorrhagic shock, cardiorespiratory arrest, pulmonary thromboembolism,

generalized seizures). Depending on their severity, duration and presumed reversibility, waiting for normalization of fetal oxygenation may be indicated. In severe situations where reversibility may take long or is uncertain, immediate delivery is warranted.

Occult and Irreversible Causes of Fetal Hypoxia

Some causes of fetal hypoxia may not be immediately identifiable (e.g., occult cord compression, fetal haemorrhage) or may not be reversible in nature (e.g., uterine rupture, placental abruption, cord prolapse). While reducing uterine contraction frequency and changing maternal position may be attempted when there is uncertainty as to the cause, prompt delivery is required when no effect is achieved of when a clearly irreversible cause is identified.

CONCLUSION

The aim of intrapartum CTG monitoring is to identify signs of reduced fetal oxygenation during labour, thereby triggering the use of appropriate obstetric interventions to avoid adverse perinatal outcomes. The

2015 FIGO guidelines constitute the largest consensus ever reached in this field. Their aims are to promote a common terminology, to improve intrapartum care throughout the world, thereby contributing to a reduction in perinatal mortality and long-term sequelae, while at the same time avoiding unnecessary obstetrical interventions. However, it remains the responsibility of healthcare professionals to understand the pathophysiology of fetal oxygenation in labour and to integrate CTG analysis into the wider clinical picture, so as to adopt the best clinical management.

REFERENCES

[1] Ayres-de-Campos D, Arulkumaran S; FIGO Intrapartum Fetal Monitoring Expert Consensus Panel. FIGO consensus guidelines on intrapartum fetal monitoring: introduction. Int J Gynecol Obstet 2015;131:3–4.

[2] Ayres-de-Campos D, Arulkumaran S; FIGO Intrapartum Fetal Monitoring Expert Consensus Panel. FIGO consensus guidelines on intrapartum fetal monitoring: physiology of fetal oxygenation and the main goals of intrapartum fetal monitoring. Int J Gynecol Obstet 2015;131:5–8.

[3] Lewis D, Downe S; FIGO Intrapartum Fetal Monitoring Expert Consensus Panel. FIGO consensus guidelines on intrapartum fetal monitoring: intermittent auscultation. Int J Gynecol Obstet 2015;131:9–12.

[4] Ayres-de-Campos D, Spong CY, Chandraharan E; FIGO Intrapartum Fetal Monitoring Expert Consensus Panel. FIGO consensus guidelines on intrapartum fetal monitoring: cardiotocography. Int J Gynecol Obstet 2015;131(1):13–24.

[5] Visser GH, Ayres-de-Campos D; FIGO Intrapartum Fetal Monitoring Expert Consensus Panel. FIGO consensus guidelines on intrapartum fetal monitoring: adjunctive technologies. Int J Gynecol Obstet 2015;131:25–9.

[6] FIGO Subcommittee on Standards in Perinatal Medicine. Guidelines for the use of fetal monitoring. Int J Gynecol Obstet 1987;25(3):159–67.

7

ANTEPARTUM FETAL SURVEILLANCE

DONALD GIBB ■ SABARATNAM ARULKUMARAN

In 2016, National Health Service (NHS) England launched a care bundle approach to reduce stillbirths.[1] The care bundle has four components based on the major contributors to stillbirths: reducing smoking in pregnancy, risk assessment and surveillance for growth restriction, raising awareness of reduced fetal movements and effective fetal monitoring during labour. This chapter deals with antenatal fetal surveillance and includes sections on detection and surveillance of growth restriction and management of reduced fetal movements.

Low-risk mothers will be seen largely by midwives in community antenatal clinics. Higher-risk mothers will be seen in hospital antenatal clinics, often by doctors. Those at risk require access to antenatal testing facilities. Maternofetal assessment units have become a standard feature in most large maternity services. The benefits of this include the gathering together of the various tests with the compilation and review of results. Daily outpatient assessment and review may be undertaken where previously hospital admission was the norm. However, easy access may result in excessive testing with largely normal results. Protocols of referral should therefore be formulated and audit undertaken. An assessment unit should be located near the ultrasound department because most testing in the antenatal period depends on ultrasound examination. The simplest method of fetal assessment is the antenatal cardiotocography (CTG). Computerized interpretation of the CTG is available from various manufacturers. These systems also provide electronic storage of the CTG; this is very useful because CTGs tend to get 'lost' and the original fades within a relatively short period of time. If a CTG is not electronically stored it

should be photocopied, as this lasts much longer. Caution should be exercised in depending on computerized trace analysis with a consequent risk of the loss of human skills of interpretation. The best computer is the human brain! The unit should be staffed by motivated midwives, who work with dedicated clinicians to assess those cases suspected to be at high risk. The individual requesting the test should be aware of the result in order to plan and justify further management. This should not be delegated by default to a junior member of staff.

IDENTIFICATION OF THE FETUS AT RISK

There are two groups of women who may require fetal assessment:

1. women with previously recognized historical risk factors such as previous stillbirth and neonatal death, or medical disorders such as diabetes mellitus, hypertension or other conditions
2. lower-risk women who develop obstetric complications during pregnancy, such as antepartum haemorrhage, hypertension, reduced fetal movement, intrauterine growth restriction (IUGR), cholestasis or prolongation of pregnancy

Adverse outcomes due to acute events like cord occlusion or placental abruption cannot be predicted by existing tests of fetal well-being. Fetal testing on account of the above markers within the past history can only be for maternal reassurance and should be minimized; excessive testing may generate anxiety and *consume much-needed resources.* Chronic compromise due to placental insufficiency operates through growth or nutritional failure of varying degrees. Some of these adverse results might be prevented by the identification of the fetus at risk and appropriate intervention. Hypoxia is not the only mechanism of compromise. Other conditions such as diabetes mellitus, Rhesus isoimmunization and maternal or fetal infection may present a different threat. The selection of tests appropriate to the condition is important. There should be a protocol for testing that is related to the condition.

Cases are referred for fetal assessment for a variety of reasons. The most common indications are an abdominal size inappropriate for gestational age and reduced fetal movements. Vaginal bleeding, preterm labour, prolongation of pregnancy and hypertension are also common.

FETAL GROWTH

The abdomen may be judged to be a different size from that expected from the dates. More commonly this is smaller rather than larger. The importance of detecting small babies in utero has been emphasized in Chapter 2.

The clinical scenario may indicate a risk of hypoxic IUGR in well-recognized situations: previous IUGR baby, malnourished mother, smoking, alcohol, drug abuse, medical conditions, gestational hypertension, multiple pregnancy and other conditions. The algorithm suggested by the Royal College of Obstetricians and Gynaecologists (RCOG) for screening and surveillance of fetal growth in singleton pregnancies is given in Figure 7.1[2] and should be used to identify mothers at risk of growth restriction. Those at low risk should have a symphysis height chart plotted and those at high risk should have serial ultrasound measurements that will provide estimated weight calculation, which should be plotted on a chart.

The measurement of the fundosymphysis height (see Figs 2.1 and 2.2) in centimetres, given that the fetus is a single fetus in a longitudinal lie, is plotted on a chart. If it is more than 2 cm smaller than the gestational age-based uterine fundal height before 36

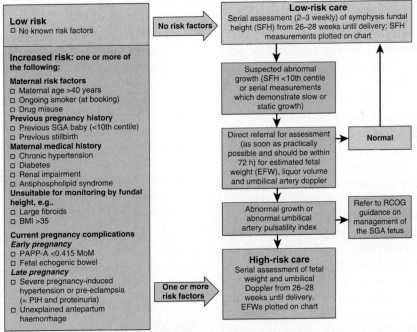

Fig. 7.1 ■ Index algorithm and risk assessment tool – screening and surveillance of fetal growth in singleton pregnancies. (Reproduced with permission from: NHS England document 'Saving Babies' lives – a Care bundle for reducing still births' – 2016 under Open Government License 3.0 and that of the Royal College of Obstetricians and Gynaecologists. *The investigation and management of small for gestational age fetus.* Green-top Guideline No. 31. London: RCOG; 2013.)

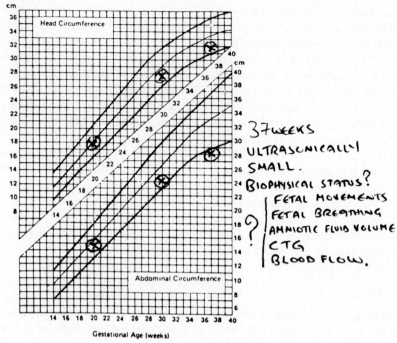

Fig. 7.2 ■ Ultrasound chart – small for dates.

weeks or 3 cm thereafter, then it is clinically small for dates. The confounding effects of abnormal lie, obesity, fibroids, multiple pregnancy and polyhydramnios must also be considered.

Clinically Small for Dates Is an Indication for an Ultrasound Scan

- On ultrasound examination measurements of head circumference (HC), abdominal circumference (AC) and femur length (FL) are taken and plotted on a growth chart (Fig. 7.2). The AC reflects fetal weight most accurately and if it falls below the 5th centile this is ultrasonically small for dates. Customized fundosymphysis fundal growth charts based on ethnicity, parity, height and weight of the mother are freely available.[3,4] They are recommended by the RCOG as they may help to identify more cases of IUGR than conventional measurements with the tape.[2] Similarly customized growth charts are available to plot estimated fetal weight based on ultrasound measurements.[3,4] A fetus that is ultrasonically small may be an

expected small but healthy baby due to small parents (i.e., genetic smallness). Alternatively, a small fetus may be pathologically small due to an abnormal process. To distinguish one from the other the following should be taken into account:

- risk factors
- amniotic fluid volume
- subjective and objective fetal movements
- CTG
- other biophysical elements: fetal breathing, fetal tone, blood flow velocity waveform in the fetal vessels by Doppler ultrasound

Pathological smallness is what is generally referred to as IUGR. This term carries an implication of a likelihood of a hypoxic process being present. The pathology of growth restriction is defined by the size, but function is more important.

Not All Small Fetuses Are Suffering From IUGR

A growth-restricted baby is one that has not realized its own intrinsic growth potential.

The growth-restricted baby identified before or on admission in labour is flagged for special care with continuous electronic fetal monitoring, careful use of oxytocic therapy when needed and no undue prolongation of the labour process. The final proof of hypoxic IUGR comes from the neonatologist's observations of weight (in relation to expected weight for gestational age) and neonatal behaviour. Usually, these babies have a scaphoid abdomen, little subcutaneous fat deposition in the limbs and can be recognized by measurement of ponderal indices.

BIOPHYSICAL ASSESSMENT OF FETAL HEALTH

Fetal Movements

From 24 weeks onward, awareness of fetal movements and their importance should be explained to every mother. Reduced or absent fetal movements should be carefully investigated using the RCOG advice[5]: perform a CTG and if there has been no scan within the last 2 weeks then also a growth scan and amniotic fluid volume assessment to exclude missed IUGR. Fetal activity in the form of fetal movement perceived by the mother is a reliable indicator of fetal health. Women should be encouraged to be aware of this. An appropriate AC and normal amniotic fluid volume on ultrasound are reassuring and often the fetus is seen to be active during the scan. The woman will also see this and be reassured. Commonly, after or even during assessment the fetus recommences normal movements and there is no need for further assessment.

In a randomized study involving 68,000 women, the routine use of fetal movement charts was not beneficial compared with more selective use.[6] Reduced or no movements predicted poor perinatal outcome but this could not be prevented. This may be partly to do with different reporting times in the study and inadequate surveillance, possibly late surveillance or being dependent only on the CTG. In order to avoid such occurrences, NHS England[1] has formulated a checklist and this is given in Box 7.1.

The commonly used chart in the UK is the Cardiff fetal movement 'Count to ten' chart. Sadovsky, who studied fetal movement extensively, suggested that there should be four fetal movements in a 2-hour (h)

BOX 7.1
CHECKLIST FOR REQUIRED MANAGEMENT OF REDUCED FETAL MOVEMENTS[a,11]

Based upon Royal College of Obstetricians and Gynaecologists Guideline No. 57.[5]
For women ≥28 weeks gestation.
Keep in guidance notes about Fetal Medicine Unit referral for women <24 weeks gestation.

ATTENDANCE WITH REDUCED FETAL MOVEMENTS (RFM)

- Ask
  Is there a maternal perception of reduced fetal movements?
- Assess
  Are there risk factors for fetal growth restriction (FGR) or stillbirth?
  Consider – multiple consultations for RFM, known FGR, maternal hypertension, diabetes, extremes of maternal age, primiparity, smoking, obesity, racial/ethnic factors, past obstetric history of FGR or stillbirth and issues with access to care.
- Act
  Auscultate fetal heart (hand-held Doppler/Pinard)
  Perform a cardiotocograph to assess fetal heart rate in accordance with national guidelines.
  If risk factors for FGR/stillbirth, perform an ultrasound scan for fetal growth, liquor volume and umbilical artery Doppler within 24 h.
- Advise
  Convey results of investigations to the mother.
  Mother should re-attend if further reductions in fetal movements at any time.
- Act
  Act upon abnormal results promptly.

[a]Reproduced with permission from: NHS England document 'Saving Babies' lives – a Care bundle for reducing still births' – 2016 under Open Government License 3.0 and that of the Royal College of Obstetricians and Gynaecologists. *Reduced Fetal Movements*, Green-top Guideline No. 57. London: RCOG; 2011.

---

period each day, of which one movement has to be strong.[7] The expectation of four fetal movements in 2 h or 10 in 12 h is arbitrary and correlates with a good perinatal outcome.[8–10] A single fetal movement felt by the mother may not be recorded by ultrasound movement detection devices. However, when a mother feels clusters of fetal movements for 15–20 seconds (s) it is detected by the ultrasound transducer and is almost always associated with fetal heart rate (FHR) accelerations.[11] Women should be encouraged to be reassured by clusters of fetal movements.

The commonest answer to the question 'Is the baby moving?' is 'Yes, a lot'. We have to be prepared for the next question 'Can it move too much? Can this be bad?' There are anecdotal reports by experienced clinicians of excessive fetal movements followed by death in utero. This must be due to an acute event and cord accidents or abruption could be postulated. In utero convulsions may occur, whether due to pre-existing brain abnormality or to another mechanism and may be reported by the mother as excessive fetal movement followed by death. In any event, it must be extremely rare and this should not compromise our general reassurance of the mother that a lot of fetal movement is a healthy phenomenon. When a woman complains of excessive fetal movements a reversion to normal movements is reassuring, but if there is a subsequent absence of fetal movement she should attend urgently for review.

Increased fetal activity can lead to a confluence of accelerations mimicking fetal tachycardia, and the synchronous automatic recording of fetal movements as done by the newest monitors will help to clarify this situation.[12] There are monitors using actograms that attempt to record fetal movement and fetal breathing in addition to the FHR. The clinical application of this principle remains to be proven, however.

Antepartum Electronic Fetal Heart Rate Monitoring

Non-Stress Test

The recording of the FHR for a period of 20–30 minutes (min) without any induced stress to the fetus (like oxytocin infusion or nipple stimulation) to produce uterine contractions is called the non-stress test (NST). In the UK this is commonly referred to as an antenatal CTG. The duration of this test should be until reactivity is observed – that is until there are two accelerations in a 10-min period. The sleep phase with no fetal movement and no FHR accelerations does not usually exceed 40 min in the vast majority of healthy fetuses and almost all healthy fetuses show a reactive trace within 90 min.[13] This forms the framework for extending the NST for 40 min when the trace is not reactive in the first 20 min.

A summary of the interpretation of the NST based on the International Federation of Obstetrics and Gynaecology (FIGO)[14,15] and the actions that are recommended with each type of trace is given below.

Antepartum Cardiotocograph (NST)

Normal/Reassuring

- At least two accelerations (15 beats for >15 s) in 10 min (reactive trace), baseline heart rate 110–150 beats per min (bpm), baseline variability 5–25 bpm, absence of decelerations.
- Sporadic mild decelerations (amplitude <40 bpm, duration <30 s) are acceptable following an acceleration.
- When there is moderate tachycardia (150–170 bpm) or bradycardia (100–110 bpm), a reactive trace without decelerations is reassuring of good health.

Interpretation/action: Repeat according to the clinical situation and the degree of fetal risk.

Suspicious/Equivocal

- Absence of accelerations for greater than 40 min (non-reactive).
- Baseline heart rate 150–170 bpm or 110–100 bpm, baseline variability greater than 25 bpm in the absence of accelerations.
- Sporadic decelerations of any type unless severe as described below.

Interpretation/action: Continue for 90 min until the trace becomes reactive, or repeat CTG within 24 h, amniotic fluid index (AFI) or single vertical pocket of amniotic fluid/biophysical profile (BPP)/Doppler ultrasound blood velocity waveform.

Pathological/Abnormal

- Baseline heart rate less than 100 bpm or greater than 170 bpm.
- Silent pattern less than 5 bpm for greater than 90 min.
- Sinusoidal pattern (oscillation frequency <2–5 cycles/min, amplitude of 2–10 bpm for >40 min with no acceleration and no area of normal baseline variability).
- Repeated late, prolonged (>1 min) and severe variable (>40 bpm) decelerations.

Interpretation/action: Further evaluation (ultrasonic assessment of amniotic fluid volume, BPP, Doppler ultrasound blood velocity waveform). Deliver if clinically appropriate.

The antepartum cardiotocograph (NST) is usually applied for diagnostic purposes; its value for screening has not been proven.[14,15] Pooled results of four studies of NSTs involving 10,169 patients revealed a satisfactory outcome with a false-negative rate of 7 per 10 000 cases.[16–19] The NST may be abnormal not only due to hypoxia but also due to other causes associated with reduced baseline variabilities such as infection, medication, congenital malformation, cerebral haemorrhage and cardiac arrhythmia. A review of the history with further evaluation will be helpful to clarify the cause.

Assessment of Amniotic Fluid Volume

Fetal urine contributes significantly to amniotic fluid volume. Fetuses with no kidneys have severe oligohydramnios. With diminished placental function and reduced renal perfusion, the amniotic fluid volume decreases. The perinatal outcome is poor when the amniotic fluid volume is reduced at delivery.[20–22]

Clinical evaluation of amniotic fluid volume by abdominal palpation can be deceptive. The impression of the amniotic fluid volume gained on ultrasound examination is fairly reliable. Objective assessment of the vertical depth of the largest pocket of amniotic fluid after excluding loops of cord or the sum of the vertical pockets in the four quadrants of the uterus (AFI) is used in practice. A recent review of the literature suggests that either AFI or the single largest vertical pocket can be used as an objective measure.[23] Reduced amniotic fluid by either method is associated with poor fetal outcome[20–22] and delivery should be considered, assuming a reasonable gestational age. If only one vertical pocket is measured, a value of less than 3 cm in the largest pool is an indication for delivery.

In post-term pregnancy or that complicated by severe growth restriction, the decline in fluid volume can be up to one-third every week, and twice-weekly assessment is advisable. Combining amniotic fluid assessment and NST could be the first-line assessments in high-risk pregnancies and is adequate for most women. Antepartum fetal death within a week of a reactive NST may occur for those who have an AFI below 5.[24] It is quite possible for a fetus with a reactive NST and good fetal movements to die suddenly in the presence of marked oligohydramnios (Fig. 7.3A–C). This may be due to umbilical cord compression. Most centres now recognize that, for high-risk pregnancies

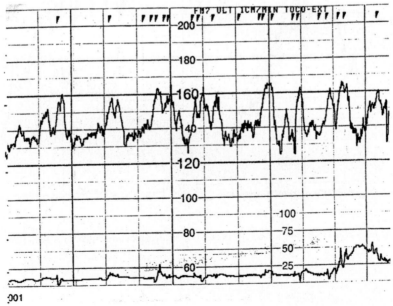

A 001

Fig. 7.3 ■ (A) Non-stress test in a post-mature fetus: variability and fetal movements seen;

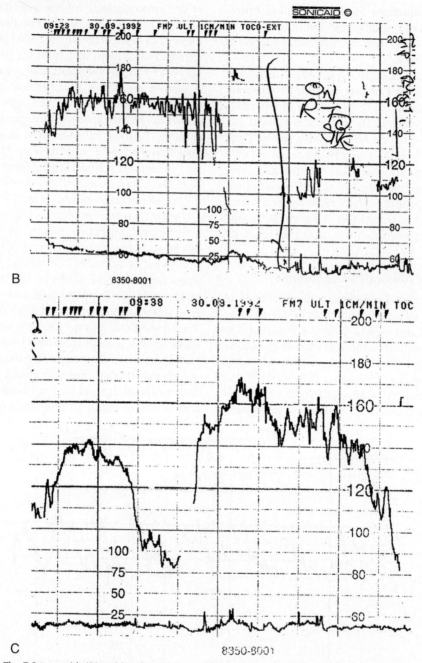

Fig. 7.3 ■ cont'd. (B) sudden decelerations; (C) bradycardia and fetal death within minutes.

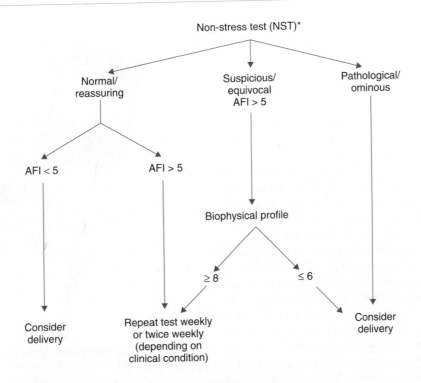

AFI; Amniotic fluid index.
*Repeat NST and AFI weekly or more often according to clinical situation.
In preterm situations additional tests (e.g., Doppler velocimetry) may be of value.

Fig. 7.4 ■ Suggestion for antepartum fetal monitoring in high-risk pregnancies.

where a reduction of amniotic fluid volume is suspected (e.g., IUGR, post-term), it is desirable to perform an amniotic fluid estimation. A schematic diagram incorporating AFI and NST as the first-line assessment is shown in Figure 7.4.

Measurement of Blood-Flow Velocity Waveforms

Sometimes it is not possible to deliver a fetus at risk of progressive hypoxia because of prematurity. There is difficulty in interpreting the NST at early gestations. Measurement of blood-flow velocity waveforms in the umbilical artery, fetal aorta, middle cerebral artery and ductus venosus may give additional useful information for the timing of delivery in these circumstances. Initially, there is increased resistance in the umbilical artery followed by reduced resistance in the middle cerebral artery. With increasing compromise, the umbilical artery Doppler may show absent or reversal of end-diastolic flow. With absent end-diastolic flow,

if the maturity does not pose a major challenge, then delivery may be undertaken. If more prolongation of the pregnancy is required then additional testing by computerized CTG or ductus venosus Doppler may be of value, the latter being preferred based on long-term outcome studies.[25] If there is a reversal of end-diastolic flow in the umbilical artery, ductus venosus flow or computerized CTG does not meet the set criteria, then it is an indication for delivery.

Biophysical Assessment

Fetal responses to hypoxia do not occur at random but rather are initiated and regulated by complex, integrated reflexes of the fetal central nervous system. Stimuli that regulate the biophysical characteristics of fetal movement, breathing and tone arise from different sites in the brain. There is some evidence that the first physical activity to develop is fetal tone at 8 weeks gestation. It is also the last to cease functioning when subjected to increasing hypoxia.[26] Fetal movements develop at 9 weeks and fetal breathing at 20 weeks. FHR activity matures last, by about 28 weeks, and is the first to be affected by hypoxia. In hypoxia, FHR characteristics may become abnormal first, followed by breathing, body and limb movements, and finally by tone.

Evaluation of more than one biophysical parameter to assess fetal health has been suggested, but it may not be necessary if the NST is reactive and amniotic fluid assessment is normal. In the assessment of BPP fetal movements, tone, breathing and amniotic fluid volume assessed by the scan and NST are considered, and for each, a score of 2 or 0 is given, there being no intermediate score.[27] When the NST is not reactive, as is more common in the preterm period, it might be useful to assess the fetal BPP. A score of 8 or 10 indicates a fetus is in good condition. Retesting should be performed at intervals depending on the level of risk. In situations where the compromise may develop faster, as in prolonged pregnancy, IUGR and pre-labour rupture of membranes, it is best performed twice weekly. If the score is 6, then the score should be re-evaluated 4–6 h later and a decision made based on the new score. When the BPP is ≤2 on one occasion, or ≤4 on two occasions (6–8 h apart), delivery of the fetus is indicated if the fetus is adequately mature and has a good chance of survival.[28] Further evaluation with fetal blood-flow velocity waveform measurement may be considered if the fetus is so premature that deferring delivery by even a few days is considered beneficial. Good perinatal outcome has been reported with BPP scoring in high-risk pregnancy[29] and as a primary modality of testing in prolonged pregnancies.[30]

A modified BPP where only the ultrasound parameters are evaluated (without NST) has been found to be equally reliable.[31] Due to the time and expertise needed to perform a BPP, many centres perform an NST and amniotic fluid assessment. Formal biophysical scoring should be reserved for fetal medicine units and research protocols.

Assessment of the Fetus in an Outpatient Clinic With Limited Facilities

A hand-held Doptone with a digital display will give a baseline FHR. New Doppler machines give a CTG on the LED screen and it is possible to identify FHR accelerations and decelerations (Fig. 7.5).

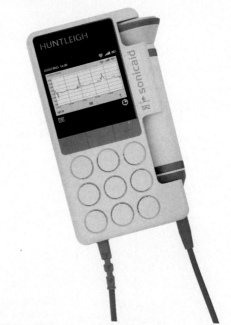

Fig. 7.5 ▮ Digital hand-held Doppler monitor with cardiac tracing. (Courtesy of Huntleigh/Sonicaid.)

NST is usually used for diagnostic purposes and has not been proven to be of value as a screening test. The ability of the test to identify the problem being investigated should be known. A normal NST indicates fetal health/well-being. However, with chronic placental dysfunction, fetal adaptation occurs and normal (reactive) NST does not indicate the degree by which placental function may be reduced. Thus, the predictive value of a normal NST is governed by the clinical situation.

CASE ILLUSTRATIONS

The CTG may not be normal owing to a variety of causes other than hypoxia: cardiac arrhythmias, heart block, brain abnormality (congenital or acquired), chromosomal abnormality, anaesthesia, drug effects and infection.

Hypoxia

Severe IUGR is seen in the preterm period. It has been suggested that decelerations are a normal feature of the preterm CTG. There is a reduction in variability, and lower-amplitude accelerations are seen in the preterm CTG (Fig. 7.6); however, major decelerations are not

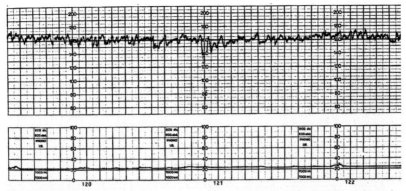

Fig. 7.6 ■ Cardiotocography in preterm baby – low-amplitude accelerations and short sharp decelerations.

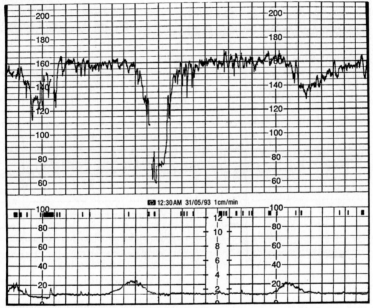

Fig. 7.7 ■ Non-stress test in a case of severe intrauterine growth restriction, oligohydramnios, poor fetal movement and abnormal fetal and poor maternal blood flow.

a normal feature. In the preterm period, short sharp decelerations of less than 15 s may be seen. They are often seen with change of state from sleeping to waking and may follow immediately after the acceleration. When major decelerations occur the clinical situation should be considered. Figure 7.7 is from a known case of severe IUGR at 25 weeks gestation. There was oligohydramnios, poor fetal movement and very abnormal fetal and maternal blood flow. On account of a very small fetal weight estimate and early gestation, the couple, with the advice of the obstetrician, opted for conservative management. The fetus died in utero 3 days later.

Given a bigger weight estimate and later gestation, delivery would have been appropriate. There will be no guarantee that the baby is not already damaged; however, there is a good chance such a baby will do well with good neonatal intensive care.[31] Leaving a fetus to die in utero is not ethically justifiable in the face of reasonable weight and gestation.

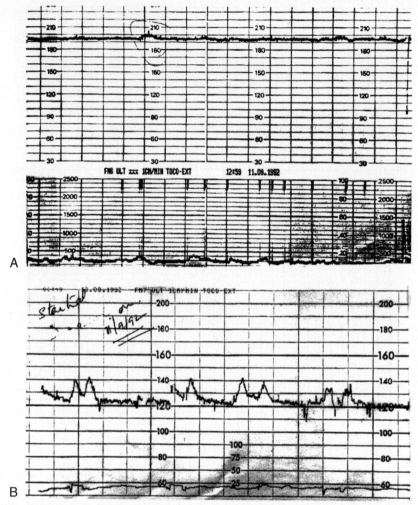

Fig. 7.8 ■ (A) Fetal supraventricular tachycardia; (B) reversal to normal rate after maternal administration of digoxin.

Cardiac Arrhythmias

Fetal arrhythmia may give rise to an abnormal trace, although the fetus is not hypoxic. Figure 7.8A was obtained from a case where the midwife auscultated the fetal heart in the antenatal clinic and heard a tachycardia. She noted that the multiparous woman was classically low risk and that the fetus was well grown and moving. This was confirmed by an ultrasound scan after referral to the hospital. Twenty hours later the CTG was repeated and was essentially unchanged. Advice was sought from a specialized unit, a diagnosis of fetal supraventricular tachycardia was made and the administration of double the adult dose of digoxin

was recommended. Fetal echocardiography was normal. Figure 7.8B was recorded the following day. The pregnancy continued, culminating in normal labour, normal intrapartum CTG and normal delivery of a healthy baby 2 weeks later. The baby had a structurally normal heart and no further problem with the heart rhythm. Figure 7.9A is a similar case but the observation of supraventricular tachycardia was made in early labour. Advice was sought and the administration of digoxin was considered inappropriate because the drug would not have taken effect until after the baby had been born. The baby was noted to be moving and continued to do so during labour. The amniotic fluid was clear and the woman was low risk. The CTG

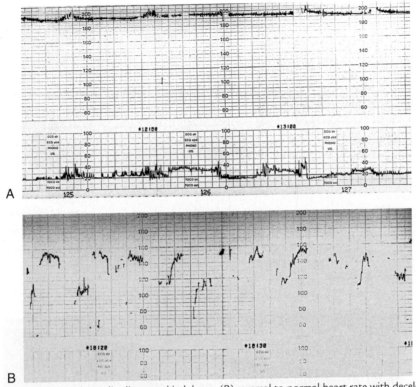

Fig. 7.9 ■ (A) Supraventricular tachycardia diagnosed in labour; (B) reversal to normal heart rate with decelerations in the second stage of labour.

remained unchanged during the 6 h of labour until the second stage. At this time the features changed, possibly due to vagal stimulation with the descent of the head. Although technically imperfect, there appeared to be a normal rate, variability and second-stage decelerations (see Fig. 7.9B). After delivery, the baby had a normal heart rate and no further problem!

Heart Block

This can be complete or partial, and continuous or intermittent. Occasional dropped beats are frequent and of no significance: they generally do not interfere with the appearance of the trace or persist after delivery. A case of maternal systemic lupus erythematosus with fetal heart block has been shown in Figure 4.27.

Brain Abnormalities – Acquired

Physiological mechanisms controlling the fetal heart require the integrity of the central nervous system.

An abnormal CTG with no accelerations or decelerations and markedly reduced baseline variability was recorded (Fig. 7.10A) when a high-risk woman on antihypertensive medication presented with a sudden cessation of fetal movement. The fetus was well grown and the amniotic fluid volume was normal on the ultrasound scan. During a prolonged scan, the fetus did not move. There was a collapsed stomach and an atonic dilated bladder with evidence of a large cerebral haemorrhage (see Fig. 7.10B). In view of the unusual findings, a fetal blood sample was obtained from the umbilical vein for karyotyping, fetal haematology and cytomegalovirus screening. The fetal blood gases were normal and the fetal haemoglobin was 8 g/dl consistent with the intracranial haemorrhage. While the karyotype results were awaited the fetus did not move and died 24 h after the procedure. Postmortem confirmed the cerebral haemorrhage. This severely 'brain-damaged' fetus was not hypoxic and, if

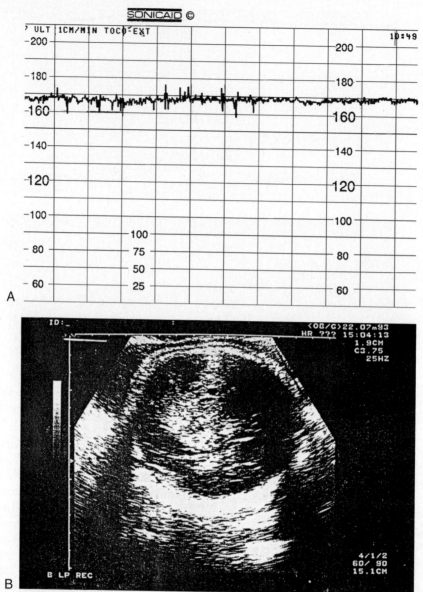

Fig. 7.10 ■ (A) Cardiotocography with a 'silent pattern' (baseline variability <5 bpm), no accelerations or decelerations; (B) scan showing evidence of fetal intracerebral haemorrhage.

delivered, would have had a very poor prognosis. The mother accepted and understood the outcome; she has since had a living child. Intracranial haemorrhage may occur in cases of alloimmune thrombocytopenia or when the woman is on warfarin therapy. When a CTG becomes abnormal despite good growth and good amniotic fluid volume, such unusual causes must be considered before deciding to deliver. Delivery will not lead to an improved outcome in these circumstances. In twin-to-twin transfusion syndrome when one fetus dies, the 'second fetus' may suffer from the consequences of sudden haemodynamic changes that may

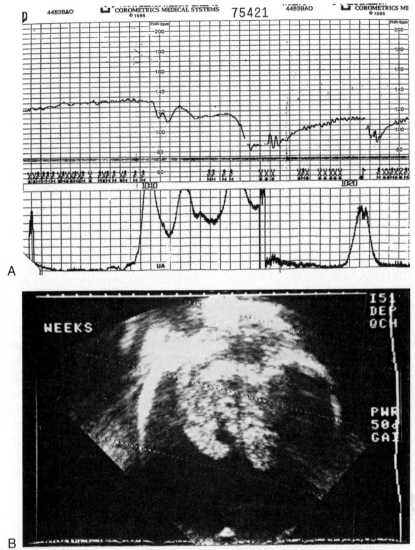

Fig. 7.11 ▪ (A) Cardiotocography: unsteady baseline heart rate but with plenty of fetal movement; (B) ultrasound scan showing the fetus with holoprosencephaly.

affect the brain and then manifest as a non-reactive CTG. No changes in blood gases on fetal blood sampling or obvious ultrasonic morphological change in the brain are seen immediately, but vacuolation in the brain may follow.

Brain Abnormalities – Congenital

The inability to maintain a steady baseline heart rate (Fig. 7.11A) can be due to severe hypoxic brain damage or may be associated with severe brain malformation.

If the fetus is active, as indicated by fetal movements, it is unlikely to be hypoxic and the cause of such a trace should be sought by further investigation. The associated pathology was holoprosencephaly, shown by ultrasound examination (see Fig. 7.11B).

Chromosomal Abnormality

A 39-year-old multiparous woman was referred from another hospital with a well-grown fetus, reduced fetal movements and a good volume of amniotic fluid, and

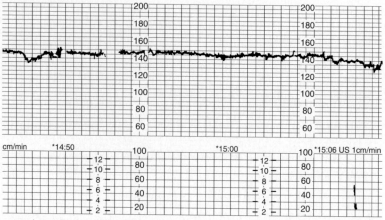

Fig. 7.12 ■ Cardiotocography with poor baseline variability, no accelerations and isolated decelerations. Misfit of fetal well-being tests; abnormal karyotype.

yet an abnormal CTG (Fig. 7.12). The Doppler blood-flow studies in the fetus and mother were normal. There was a slightly reduced FL and slight hydrone-phrosis. Delivery was deferred until the result of karyo-type from a fetal blood sample was known. The fetus died in utero the day before the result, showing Down syndrome, became available. The mother had been counselled of this strong possibility and requested that the baby not be delivered without the karyotype result.

In chromosomally abnormal fetuses, especially trisomies, the central neural pathway may be disorga-nized resulting in an abnormal CTG,[32] although the fetal growth, amniotic fluid volume and fetal move-ments may be normal. In trisomy 13 and 18, the fetus might be growth restricted with an increased amniotic fluid volume. In a proportion of these cases the CTG shows a steady baseline but with poor baseline vari-ability, reduced or absent accelerations and isolated decelerations. The disorganized neural development may manifest after birth as neurodevelopmental delay.

A misfit of fetal function tests suggests the need for further investigations.

Fetal Anaemia

This may show a sinusoidal or sinusoidal-like pattern and is discussed in Chapter 11.

Anaesthesia

The fetus is anaesthetized as well as the mother! The fetus may excrete the drugs more slowly than the mother. A multiparous woman fractured her tibia at 29 weeks gestation. She was given a general anaesthetic in order to insert a pin and plate. A CTG performed on her return from the operating theatre 2 h after induc-tion of anaesthesia showed a dramatic reduction of baseline variability and the absence of accelerations (Fig. 7.13A). The inexperienced junior doctor sus-pected hypoxia and thought delivery might be neces-sary. An ultrasound scan confirmed a well-grown fetus and reasonable amniotic fluid volume. The consultant recommended a repeat CTG 2 h later (see Fig. 7.13B) and another 24 h after that (see Fig. 7.13C). The preg-nancy progressed normally to term without further complications.

Drug Effects

Sedatives, tranquilizers, anti-hypertensives and other drugs that act on the central nervous system tend to reduce the amplitude of the accelerations and suppress the baseline variability. In these situations, other forms of surveillance become necessary. With antihyperten-sive therapy, fetal activity may be unaffected. Cortico-steroids given to achieve fetal lung maturity can also reduce the baseline variability for 24–48 h.

Infections

A fetal tachycardia associated with a maternal infec-tion is a cause for concern. The mechanism may be a direct fetal infection or secondary response of the fetus due to the transplacental passage of pyrogens or

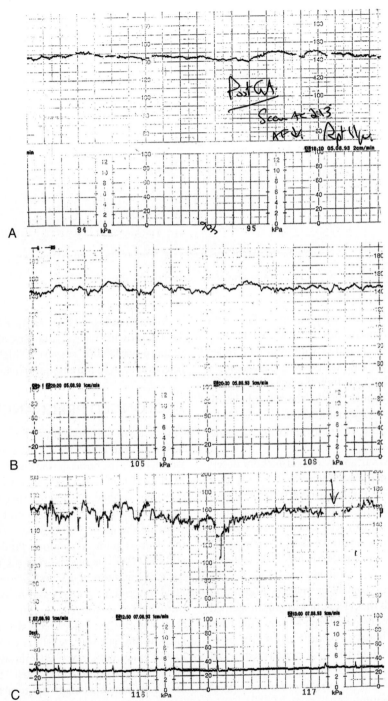

Fig. 7.13 ■ (A) Cardiotocography (CTG) performed 2 h after induction of anaesthesia: no accelerations and reduced baseline variability; (B) CTG 4 h after induction of anaesthesia; (C) CTG 24 h later – reactive trace after the effect of anaesthesia has worn off.

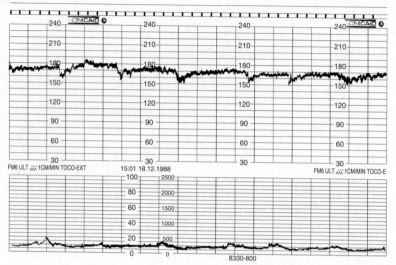

Fig. 7.14 ■ Ominous trace – listerial infection.

adrenergic metabolites. When fetal tachycardia occurs with maternal tachycardia due to maternal urinary tract infection, it usually settles with antibiotic treatment. However, when fetal tachycardia persists for a considerable period of time then the fetus may not be able to tolerate it. Consideration of the clinical picture will suggest whether an actual fetal infection is likely. Preservation of baseline variability and reactivity suggests a resilient fetus.

If there is reduced variability with or without decelerations in the absence of accelerations, the fetus itself is sick. A mother was admitted with a systemic illness at 33 weeks gestation and tachycardia. On assumption of the diagnosis of urinary tract infection, a cephalosporin was prescribed. The trace showed tachycardia with markedly reduced variability and shallow decelerations (Fig. 7.14). The mother's condition did not improve, nor did the fetal heart tracing. Rupture of the membranes with the release of meconium-stained amniotic fluid prompted caesarean section. The baby succumbed within hours of birth to congenital listeriosis; it was heavily infected. This is reflected in the seriously abnormal fetal heart tracing.

Maternal illness and preterm meconium suggest possible listerial infection.

Suspicion of the diagnosis, blood cultures and treatment with ampicillin might have led to a better outcome.[33]

In cases with prelabour rupture of the membranes, a CTG showing tachycardia, lack of accelerations and reduced variability suggest a higher probability of infection even in the absence of clinical signs.

PROLONGED PREGNANCY

This is a common indication for assessment in many hospitals. The clinician will have reviewed the menstrual and ultrasound dating and most cases will have reached 41 weeks. The CTG may be normal but caution should be applied in being reassured by this. Figure 7.3 was obtained in the assessment unit in a case where the maturity was 42 weeks and 5 days. Two days previously the deepest pool of amniotic fluid had been 3.2 cm and the CTG was reactive. On the day of assessment, the CTG was the first investigation to be performed. Fetal movements are seen on the trace and the first 7 min suggest reasonable baseline variability although at a slightly fast rate. Deep decelerations followed and the woman was transferred to the labour ward. In the anaesthetic room 20 min after the end of the trace, an ultrasound scan showed a terminal bradycardia. A decision was made not to deliver and the heart stopped within minutes of observation. The baby was found to be otherwise normal at postmortem examination. Again the presentation suggests possible cord compression with oligohydramnios as the mechanism.

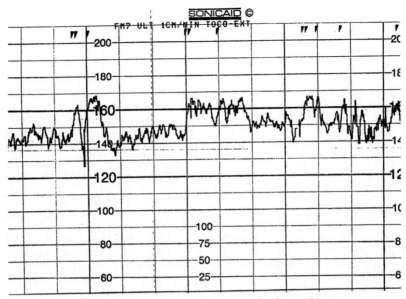

Fig. 7.15 ■ Postmature intrauterine death next day.

In another case where intrauterine death occurred 24 h after a CTG in a postmature gestation (Fig. 7.15), the CTG had been normal and a single deepest pool of amniotic fluid had been 2 cm. Since that case, we have performed AFI measurement during an assessment. In recent years the risks of fetal compromise in post-EDD gestation particularly in the older mother have been more widely appreciated. Such cases usually proceed to planned delivery before 41 weeks.

Amniotic fluid assessment should form an integral part of an assessment of fetal well-being.

REFERENCES

[1] NHS England. Saving babies' lives. Online. Available: https://www.england.nhs.uk/wp-content/uploads/2016/03/saving-babies-lives-car-bundl.pdf. [accessed 10 Aug 2016].

[2] Royal College of Obstetricians and Gynaecologists (RCOG). The investigation and management of the small-for-gestational-age fetus. Green-top Guideline No. 31. 2nd ed. Feb 2013; minor revisions Jan 2014. London: RCOG. Online. Available: https://www.rcog.org.uk/globalassets/documents/guidelines/gtg_31.pdf. [accessed 10 Aug 2016].

[3] Growth charts. Gestation Network. Online. Available: http://www.gestation.net/growthcharts.htm. [accessed 10 Aug 2016].

[4] National Health Service (NHS). Grow-AC. Antenatal charts – for antenatal plotting of fundal height and estimated fetal weight. Online. Available: http://www.perinatal.nhs.uk/growth/grow%20documentation.pdf. [accessed 10 Aug 2016].

[5] Royal College of Obstetricians and Gynaecologists (RCOG). Reduced fetal movements. Green-top Guideline No. 57. February 2011. Online. Available: https://www.rcog.org.uk/globalassets/documents/guidelines/gtg_57.pdf. [accessed 10 Aug 2016].

[6] Grant A, Elbourne D, Valentin L, et al. Routine formal fetal movement counting and risk of antepartum late death in normally formed singletons. Lancet 1989;2(8659):345–9.

[7] Sadovsky E, Yaffe H, Polishuk WZ. Fetal movements in pregnancy and urinary estriol in prediction of impending fetal death in utero. Isr J Med Sci 1974;10:1096–9.

[8] Sadovsky E, Yaffe H. Daily fetal movement recording and fetal prognosis. Obstet Gynecol 1973;41:845–50.

[9] Sadovsky E. Monitoring fetal movement: a useful screening test. Cont Obstet Gynaecol 1985;25:123–7.

[10] Sadovsky E, Rabinowitz R, Yaffe H. Decreased fetal movements and fetal malformations. J Foetal Med 1981;1:62–4.

[11] Fai F, Singh K, Malcus P, Malcus P, et al. Assessment of fetal health should be based on maternal perception of clusters rather than episodes of fetal movements. J Obstet Gynaecol Res 1996;22:299–304.

[12] Stanco LM, Rabello Y, Medearis AL, et al. Does Doppler-detected fetal movement decrease the incidence of nonreactive nonstress tests? Obstet Gynecol 1993;82:999–1003.

[13] Patrick J, Carmichael L, Laurie C, et al. Accelerations of the human fetal heart rate at 38 to 40 weeks' gestational age. Am J Obstet Gynecol 1984;148:35–41.

[14] International Federation of Obstetrics and Gynaecology (FIGO). Guidelines for the use of fetal monitoring. Int J Gynecol Obstet 1987;25:159–67.

[15] Ayres-de-Campos D, Spong CY, Chandraharan E, International Federation of Obstetrics and Gynaecology (FIGO). FIGO consensus guidelines on intrapartum fetal monitoring: cardiotocography. Int J Gynecol Obstet 2015;131(1):13–24. Online. Available: http://www.ijgo.org/article/S0020-7292(15)00395-1/pdf. [accessed 10 Aug 2016].

[16] Kubli F, Boos R, Ruttgers H, et al. Antepartum fetal heart rate monitoring and ultrasound in obstetrics. In: Beard RW, editor. Royal College of obstetricians and Gynaecologists (RCOG) Scientific meeting. London: RCOG; 1977. p. 28–47.

[17] Schifrin BS, Foye G, Amato J, et al. Routine fetal heart rate monitoring in the antepartum period. Obstet Gynecol 1979;54:21–5.

[18] Keagan Jr KA, Paul RH. Antepartum fetal heart rate testing. IV. The nonstress test as a primary approach. Am J Obstet Gynecol 1980;136:75–80.

[19] Flynn AM, Kelly J, Mansfield H, et al. A randomized controlled trial of non-stress antepartum cardiotocography. Br J Obstet Gynaecol 1982;89:427–33.

[20] Chamberlain PF, Manning FA, Morrison I, et al. Ultrasound evaluation of amniotic fluid volume. I. The relationship of marginal and decreased amniotic fluid volumes to perinatal outcome. Am J Obstet Gynecol 1984;150:245–9.

[21] Crowley P, O'Herlihy C, Boylon P. The value of ultrasound measurement of amniotic fluid volume in the management of prolonged pregnancies. Br J Obstet Gynaecol 1984;91:444–5.

[22] Morris RK, Meller CH, Tamblyn J, et al. Association and prediction of amniotic fluid measurements for adverse pregnancy outcome: systematic review and meta-analysis. BJOG 2014;121(6):686–99. https://doi.org/10.1111/1471-0528.12589.

[23] Sande JA, Ioannou C, Sarris I, et al. Reproducibility of measuring amniotic fluid index and single deepest vertical pool throughout gestation. Prenat Diagn 2015;35(5):434–9. https://doi.org/10.1002/pd.4504.

[24] Anandakumar C, Biswas A, Arulkumaran S, et al. Should assessment of amniotic fluid volume form an integral part of antenatal fetal surveillance of high risk pregnancy? Aust N Z J Obstet Gynaecol 1993;33:272–5.

[25] Lees CC, Marlow N, van Wassenaer-Leemhuis A, et al. 2 year neurodevelopmental and intermediate perinatal outcomes in infants with very preterm fetal growth restriction (TRUFFLE): a randomised trial. Lancet 2015;385(9983):2162–72. https://doi.org/10.1016/S0140-6736(14)62049-3.

[26] Vintzileos AM, Fleming AD, Scorza WE, et al. Relationship between fetal biophysical activities and umbilical cord blood gas values. Am J Obstet Gynecol 1991;165:707–12.

[27] Manning FA, Platt LD, Sipos L. Antepartum fetal evaluation: development of a fetal biophysical profile. Am J Obstet Gynecol 1980;136:787–90.

[28] Manning FA, Morrison I, Harman CR, et al. Fetal assessment based on fetal biophysical profile scoring: experience in 19,221 referred high-risk pregnancies. II. An analysis of false-negative fetal deaths. Am J Obstet Gynecol 1987;157:880–4.

[29] Johnson JM, Hareman CR, Lange IR, et al. Biophysical profile scoring in the management of the postterm pregnancy: an analysis of 307 patients. Am J Obstet Gynecol 1986;154:269–73.

[30] Eden RD, Seifert LS, Koack LD, et al. A modified biophysical profile for antenatal fetal surveillance. Obstet Gynecol 1988;71:365–9.

[31] Drew JH, Kelly E, Chew FT, et al. Prospective study of the quality of survival of infants with critical fetal reserve detected by antenatal cardiotocography. Aust N Z J Obstet Gynaecol 1992;32:32–5.

[32] Navot D, Mor-Yosef S, Granat M, et al. Antepartum fetal heart rate pattern associated with major congenital malformations. Obstet Gynecol 1983;63:414–7.

[33] Buchdahl R, Hird M, Gibb D, et al. Listeriosis revisited: the role of the obstetrician. Br J Obstet Gynaecol 1990;97:186–9.

8

THE ADMISSION TEST BY CARDIOTOCOGRAPHY OR BY AUSCULTATION

SABARATNAM ARULKUMARAN ▪ DONALD GIBB

The 2014 National Institute for Health and Care Excellence (NICE) guideline 'Intrapartum care for healthy women and their babies' states (points 1.4.6–1.4.10): 'Auscultate the fetal heart rate at first contact with the woman in labour, and at each further assessment. Auscultate the fetal heart rate for a minimum of 1 minute immediately after a contraction and record it as a single rate. Palpate the maternal pulse to differentiate between maternal heart rate and fetal heart rate. Record accelerations and decelerations if heard. Do not perform cardiotocography (CTG) on admission for low-risk women in suspected or established labour in any birth setting as part of the initial assessment.'[1] The Birthplace UK (2011) study indicates that the incidence of stillbirths after the start of care in labour is 0.22/1000, that of the death of the baby in the first week of life is 0.28/1000 and that of neonatal encephalopathy is 1.6/1000.[2] With such low figures of adverse outcome the numbers that need to be studied to evaluate whether an admission CTG could be useful will run into several thousand. Based on available data, we do not have sufficient data to state that admission CTG should not be performed. In several hospitals in Nordic countries, with a very low intrapartum fetal death rate, admission CTG is routine. We believe that the choice should be given to the mother after giving her the available information including that no definitive benefit is known and also that it increases the obstetric intervention rate. However, this debate could be resolved with the availability of graphic Doppler which shows the baseline rate, variability, accelerations and decelerations (see Ch.3). The baseline rate is best obtained when there are no contractions or fetal movements; accelerations by listening at the time of fetal movements and decelerations by listening during and soon after the contractions.

Fetal morbidity and mortality are greater in high-risk women with hypertension, diabetes, intrauterine growth restriction (IUGR) and other risk factors. A greater number of antenatal deaths are observed in this group. In pregnancies that have proceeded to term, morbidity and mortality due to events in labour occur with similar frequency in those categorized as low risk compared with those categorized as high risk based on traditional risk classification.[3,4] This may be because high-risk cases such as intrauterine growth restriction have been missed during antenatal care. To resolve this we have to turn our attention to better screening during the antenatal period and at the onset of labour. As stated above, the fetal heart rate (FHR) is auscultated after admission and every 15 min for a period of 1 min after a contraction in the first stage of labour and every 5 min or after every other contraction in the second stage of labour. During auscultation, the baseline FHR can be measured, but other features of the FHR such as baseline variability, accelerations and decelerations are more difficult to observe and quantify unless a graphic display Doppler is used or the following recommendation about auscultation is adhered to.

ADMISSION TEST BY AUSCULTATION ('INTELLIGENT AUSCULTATION')

If we are to limit our practice to auscultation it would be useful to use a Doptone so that the mother and her partner can listen. This is a very important part of their experience and they should be involved. On admission, the mother must be asked the question as to when the baby moved last and the time noted. A baseline FHR can be taken and recorded. With her permission, the midwife or doctor could place a hand on the maternal abdomen and ask the mother to notify the examiner when she feels the baby moving. The caregiver can note that he/she felt the fetal movements along with the mother, and auscultation at this time showed a rise in the FHR of 15 beats more than the baseline heart rate as accelerations are expected with fetal movements. The mother should be asked to indicate when she starts feeling a uterine contraction. The caregiver should palpate the uterine contraction and listen to the FHR during and soon after the contraction. The presence or absence of decelerations and whether recovery back to the baseline rate was after the end of the contraction should be noted. Decelerations that outlast the contractions are likely to be atypical variable or late decelerations and warrant repeat auscultation during the next two contractions and to make a decision whether further surveillance should be by continuous CTG.

If fetal movements are felt, the FHR acceleration is heard with the fetal movement, and there is no deceleration with, or soon after, a contraction, then the examiner can reassure the mother of good fetal health. Subsequent observations should be as recommended (i.e. to listen every 15 min for 1 min soon after a contraction in the first stage and after every 5 min in the second stage of labour). Non-technological monitoring is undertaken during home births by competent midwives using this principle.

Figure 4.31 shows an admission CTG of a distressed fetus with a pathological trace. Auscultation after a contraction by a skilled midwife (indicated by black dots) showed a 'normal' heart rate of 150 beats per min (bpm).

Baseline Variability Is Not Audible to the Unaided Ear

The features that will provide reassurance of fetal health are the presence of accelerations, normal baseline variability and an absence of decelerations that outlasts the contractions.

An admission test (AT) should pick up the apparently low-risk woman whose fetus is compromised on admission or is likely to become compromised in labour. This admission test may be performed by a CTG or by graphic Doppler or by 'intelligent' auscultation correlating the FHR observations to clinical events of fetal movements and contractions.

The AT by CTG (i.e., a short) continuous electronic FHR recording immediately on admission gives a better impression of the fetal condition compared with simple auscultation. In many hospitals, electronic monitoring is performed but it is done long after admission. The mother may have waited for a bed, a nightdress, general observations to be noted and other administrative issues to be resolved. In most instances, the mother walking into the labour ward is entirely healthy and her main concern is to have a healthy baby. An AT may identify those who are already at risk with an ominous pattern on admission even without any contractions (Fig. 8.1). In those with a normal or suspicious FHR the functional stress of the uterine contractions in early labour may bring about the abnormal FHR changes (Fig. 8.2). These changes may be subtle and difficult to identify by auscultation. A careful review may reveal a reduced fundosymphysis height (FSH) with a growth-restricted fetus in such cases. An admission CTG can be considered to function in the same way as a natural oxytocin challenge test.

STUDIES ON ADMISSION CARDIOTOCOGRAPHY

In Kandang Kerbau Hospital in Singapore, a blinded AT study was carried out on 1041 low-risk women.[5] A FHR tracing was obtained after covering the digital display of the FHR and the recording paper and turning down the volume so that the research midwife had no information about what the FHR trace was showing. The transducer was adjusted based on the green signal light of a fetal monitor (Hewlett-Packard 8040 or 8041), which indicates good signal quality and produces a good tracing. The trace, obtained for 20 min immediately on admission, was sealed in an envelope and put aside for later analysis. These women were a low-risk population based on risk factors and hence were sent to the low-risk labour ward for care by

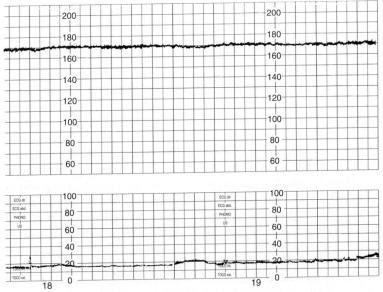

Fig. 8.1 ■ Abnormal admission test without contractions.

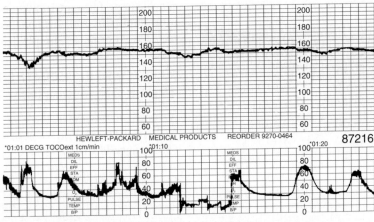

Fig. 8.2 ■ Contraction stress is often present in an admission test.

intermittent auscultation. This study was accepted by the departmental ethical committee because the normal practice at that time was that none of the low-risk women had any electronic monitoring.

For this study, a reactive normal FHR trace was defined as a recording with normal baseline rate and variability, two accelerations of 15 beats above the baseline for 15 s, and no decelerations. A 'suspicious' or 'equivocal' trace was one that had no accelerations in addition to one abnormal feature such as reduced baseline variability (<5 bpm), presence of decelerations, baseline tachycardia or bradycardia. A trace was classified as 'ominous' when more than one abnormal feature or repeated atypical variable or late decelerations were present. To evaluate the outcome, 'fetal distress' was considered to be present when ominous FHR changes led to a caesarean section or forceps delivery, or if the newborn had an Apgar score less than 7 at 5 min after spontaneous delivery (Table 8.1).

In women with ominous ATs ($n = 10$), 40% developed fetal distress compared with 1.4% (13 out of 982) in those with a reactive AT. Of those 13 who developed fetal distress after a reactive AT, 10 did so more than 5 h after the AT. Of the three who developed fetal distress in less than 5 h, one had cord prolapse (baby born by caesarean section in good condition) and the other two fetuses were less than 35 weeks gestation. They had low Apgar scores at birth 3 and 4 h after the AT but needed minimal resuscitation. In those with an ominous AT there was one fresh stillbirth of a normally formed baby with normal birth weight for gestational age at term. The midwife was charting the FHR as 140/min every 20 min for 2 h when she reported that she was unable to hear the FHR. The admission test trace is shown in Figure 8.3. There is no doubt that the midwife's observations were correct; but unfortunately, she could not hear the poor baseline variability and the shallow decelerations, which are ominous features, although the baseline rate was normal.

Barring acute events, the AT may be a good predictor of fetal condition at the time of admission and during the next few hours of labour in term fetuses labelled as low risk. If the AT is normal and reactive, gradually developing hypoxia will be reflected by no accelerations, onset of decelerations that increase in depth and duration with the progress of time and by a gradually rising baseline FHR; the latter could be picked up at the time of intermittent auscultation or electronic monitoring. Figure 8.4A–F shows sequential changes in **'gradually developing hypoxia'** in an 8-h labour showing onset of decelerations that progressively show an increase in depth and duration, reduction in the inter-deceleration interval and gradual rise of FHR with absent accelerations and reduction of baseline variability with the progress of time. A study has shown that in a well-grown fetus with clear amniotic fluid and a reactive trace if it starts to develop an abnormal FHR pattern it takes some time with these FHR changes before acidosis develops. It was estimated that, in these situations, for 50% of the babies to become acidotic took 115 min with repeated late decelerations, 145 min with repeated variable decelerations and 185 min with a flat trace.[6] Therefore, it can be safely assumed that if the AT was reactive it is reasonable to perform intermittent auscultation. In some institutions, this is further enhanced by 20 min of electronic monitoring 2–3-hourly in low-risk labour.

RANDOMIZED CONTROLLED TRIALS ON ADMISSION TEST

A systematic review of three randomized controlled trials ($n = 11,259$) and 11 observational studies ($n = 5831$) suggests that there is no evidence to support

TABLE 8.1

Results of Admission Test in Relation to the Incidence of 'Fetal Distress'

	Admission Test	Fetal Distress
Reactive	$n = 982$ (94.3%)	13 (1.4%)
Equivocal	$n = 49$ (4.7%)	5 (10.0%)
Ominous	$n = 10$ (1.0%)	4 (40.0%)§

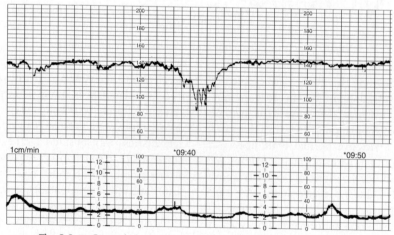

Fig. 8.3 ■ Concealed admission test of a fetus who died intrapartum.

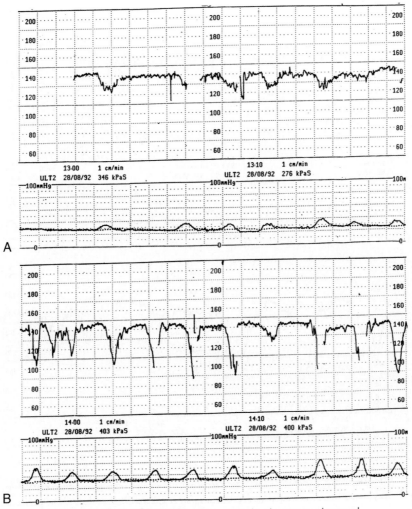

Fig. 8.4 ■ (A–F) Sequential cardiotocography changes to abnormal.

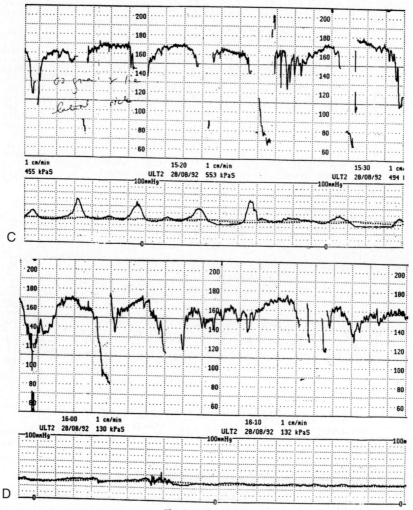

Fig. 8.4 ▪ cont'd

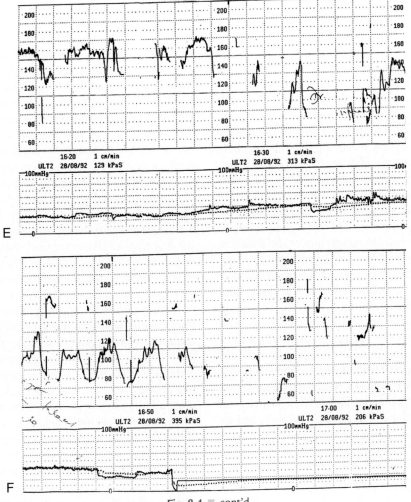

Fig. 8.4 ■ cont'd

the labour admission test.[7] The two large randomized controlled trials[8,9] did not show any benefit in terms of neonatal outcome.

In those who had the admission CTG, the epidural analgesia rate was increased (relative risk [RR] 1.35; 95% confidence interval [CI] 1.1–1.4), as well as the incidence of continuous electronic fetal monitoring (EFM) (RR 1.3; 95% CI 1.2–1.5) and fetal blood sampling (FBS) (RR 1.3; 95% CI 1.1–1.5). The operative delivery rate was the same in the two groups, suggesting that this may have been due to the increased fetal scalp blood-sampling rate in those who had the admission CTG. The study from Dublin[9] contributed 8580 out of the total of 11,259 cases for this meta-analysis.[7] In the Dublin study,[9] the presence of clear amniotic fluid was a prerequisite to enter the study. In order to achieve this, artificial rupture of membranes was performed at a mean cervical dilatation of 1.2 cm. This may not be an acceptable practice in many centres. We believe that the latter study influenced the outcome of the meta-analysis. There were higher rates of continuous EFM and a higher incidence of FBS, and this may be because, in this study, 32% of admission CTGs were considered suspicious or abnormal – an unexpectedly high percentage in early labour in women with clear amniotic fluid. Despite no definitive evidence to support admission CTG, it is carried out in many units and the CTG not discontinued, and we believe that this may be due to a lack of confidence in the interpretation of the CTG or to the shortage of midwives to provide one-to-one care, including auscultation every 15 min as recommended by NICE.[1]

OTHER FORMS OF ADMISSION TEST

The amniotic fluid index (AFI) and Doppler indices of umbilical artery blood flow, to assess fetal well-being in early labour, have been evaluated as useful screening tests for fetal distress in labour.[10,11] However, these tests need expensive equipment and expertise compared with an admission CTG which is currently simplified by the availability of graphic display Doppler devices (see Ch. 3).

ASSESSMENT OF AMNIOTIC FLUID VOLUME

Perinatal mortality and morbidity are increased in the presence of reduced amniotic fluid volume at delivery.[12,13] A reproducible semiquantitative measurement of amniotic fluid volume in early labour could conceivably be used as an adjunct to an admission CTG to triage a fetus to a high- or low-risk status in early labour.[14] In a study involving 120 women in early labour, it was found that ultrasound measurement of the vertical depth of two amniotic fluid pockets could be easily and rapidly performed by medical and midwifery staff and that the results were easily reproducible.[15] It found that a vertical depth of two pools of amniotic fluid over 3 cm was highly sensitive and predictive when used as a predictor of the absence of significant fetal distress in the first stage of labour. In this study, six women had a vertical depth of less than 3 cm; four of these women had a caesarean section in the first stage of labour for fetal distress, and in three of the newborns the cord pH was less than 7.2. None of the women who had amniotic fluid volume greater than 3 cm required caesarean section for fetal distress. In a study of 1092 singleton pregnancies,[16] amniotic fluid volume was 'quantified' by measuring the AFI, using the four-quadrant technique.[17] An AFI of less than 5 in early labour, even in the presence of a normal admission CTG, was associated with higher operative delivery rates for fetal distress, low Apgar scores, more infants needing assisted ventilation and a higher admission rate to the neonatal intensive care unit. When the admission CTG was suspicious, an AFI of greater than 5 was associated with better obstetric outcomes compared with those with an AFI of less than 5. A low AFI of below 5 may indicate incipient hypoxia and the stress of cord compression or gradual decline of oxygenation with contractions in labour may be the cause of poor outcome.

Umbilical Artery Doppler Velocimetry

Umbilical artery Doppler velocimetry has been used as an admission test. However, it has been shown to be a poor predictor of fetal distress in labour in the low-risk population.[10,18] A study of 1092 women has shown Doppler velocimetry on admission to be of little value in the presence of a normal admission CTG. However, in cases with a suspicious admission CTG, normal Doppler velocimetry was associated with fewer operative deliveries for fetal distress, better Apgar scores and less need for assisted ventilation or admission to the neonatal intensive care unit.[16]

RELATIONSHIP OF NEUROLOGICALLY IMPAIRED TERM INFANTS TO RESULTS OF ADMISSION TEST

There is controversy regarding the value of continuous EFM, let alone an admission test. Other than acute or terminal patterns of prolonged bradycardia or prolonged decelerations of a large amplitude and duration, there is little information regarding FHR patterns and neurological handicap at term[19–22] other than some observation of neurological impairment and non-reactivity,[23–25] especially in the presence of meconium. In an investigation of 48 neurologically impaired singleton term infants, the admission FHR findings and the FHR patterns 30 min before delivery were analysed.[26] Findings of this investigation are shown in Tables 8.2 and 8.3.

Based on the data in Tables 8.2 and 8.3, it is clear that fetuses with a reactive AT (accelerations) will show the following features prior to or when becoming hypoxic: all will exhibit decelerations (100%);

TABLE 8.2

Admission FHR Findings in 48 Neurologically Impaired Term Infants Separated on the Basis of FHR Reactivity[26]

FHR Pattern on Admission up to 120 min	Reactive (n = 15)	Non-Reactive (n = 33)
FHR variability (average)	14 (93%)	12[a] (36%)
Decelerations	2 (13%)	27 (82%)
Tachycardia	0 (0%)	6 (18%)

[a]$P < 0.001$.

TABLE 8.3

FHR Pattern in the Last 30 min Before Delivery, Separated on the Basis of Admission FHR Pattern[26]

Admission FHR Pattern Last 30 min Before Delivery	Reactive (n = 15)	Non-Reactive (n = 33)
FHR variability (average)	1 (7%)	11[a] (33%)
Decelerations	15 (100%)	5 (15%)
Tachycardia	14 (93%)	9[b] (27%)

[a]$P < 0.05$.
[b]$P < 0.001$.

almost all will have reduced baseline variability (93%) and tachycardia (93%). The one case where the FHR did not exceed 160 bpm showed an increase in the baseline rate by 25% and decelerations, which can be picked up on auscultation and action taken. On the other hand, if the AT is non-reactive the development of further abnormal features with the progress of labour are variable and subtle; this is difficult to recognize by intermittent auscultation. This is because already there might have been hypoxic damage and the fetus is unable to respond. In those with a non-reactive AT, nearly 82% had decelerations on the AT and 64% had reduced baseline variability (below 5 bpm) and many (82%) had a normal baseline rate. The fact that a hypoxic fetus can have a normal baseline rate and shallow decelerations of less than 15 bpm in a non-reactive trace when the baseline variability is below 5 bpm is not widely appreciated (see Fig. 8.3).

All fetuses who exhibited a reactive AT had decelerations and a gradually increasing baseline FHR suggestive of developing fetal hypoxia. It is not difficult to identify decelerations and increases in baseline FHR on auscultation (see Fig. 13.6A–J). A randomized study compared the obstetric outcome in a group who had intermittent auscultation and 2-hourly 20 min of CTG following the admission test with a group who had continuous EFM.[27] The obstetric outcome, in terms of operative delivery, low Apgar scores and admission to the neonatal unit, was the same in the two groups. The interval between admission to the labour ward to first detected FHR abnormality was the same in the two groups. This finding reassures that FHR can be confidently auscultated for changes that will indicate 'fetal distress' if the AT showed a reactive trace. On the other hand, if the trace was non-reactive with a silent pattern (baseline variability below 5) for over 90 min with shallow or no decelerations, the fetus may already be compromised or is likely to become compromised. Action should be taken to establish the acid-base status by FBS, or delivery should be considered based on the clinical scenario, e.g. absent fetal movements, infection, IUGR, meconium or post term. Failure to take action may end in fetal death (Fig. 8.5A–J). It is difficult to know whether the fetus is already hypoxic or acidotic or is suffering from another insult (e.g., infection, brain injury due to haemorrhage) unless the acid-base status is known prior to or after delivery. Cases with

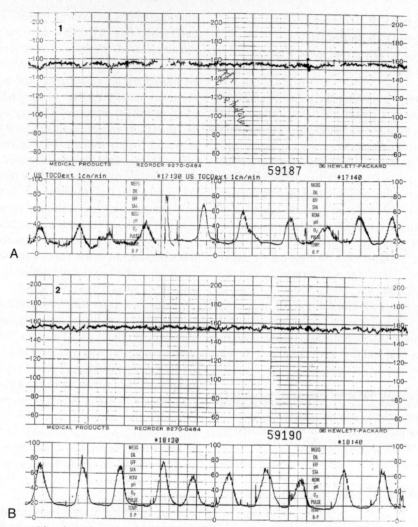

Fig. 8.5 ■ (A–J) A trace with reduced baseline variability for greater than 90 min is abnormal, especially in the presence of shallow decelerations in a non-reactive trace. Sequential traces until the baby's demise are shown.

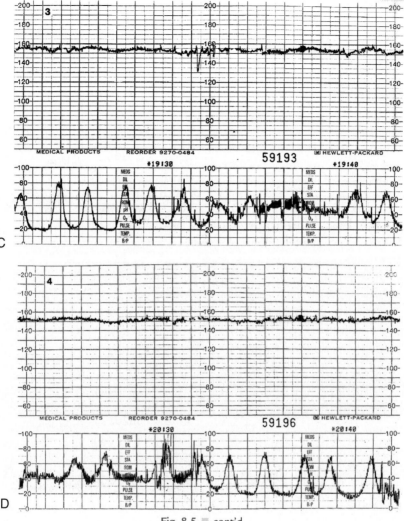

Fig. 8.5 ■ cont'd

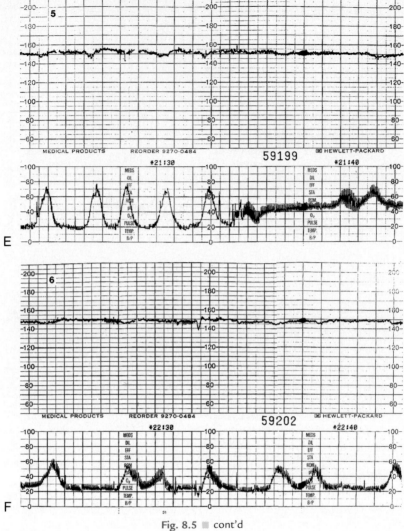

Fig. 8.5 ▪ cont'd

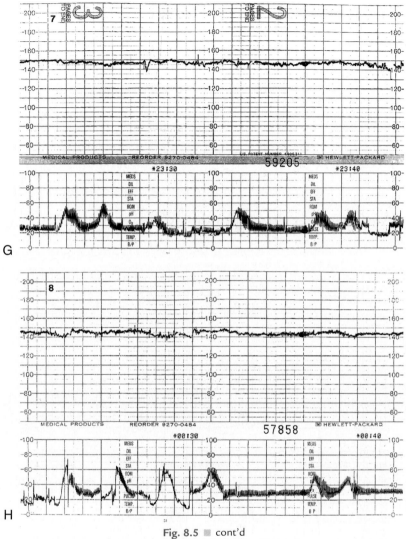

Fig. 8.5 ▪ cont'd

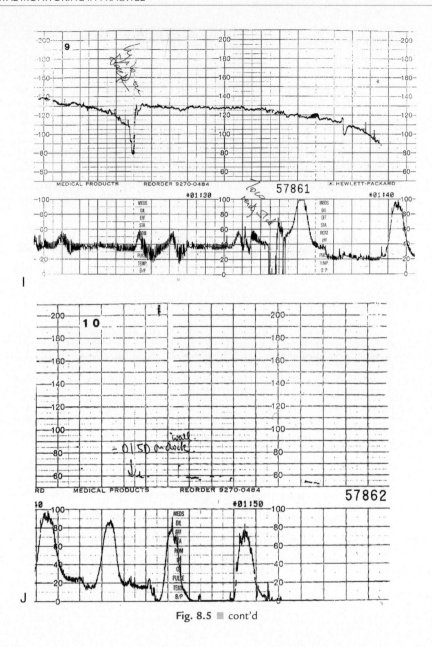

Fig. 8.5 ■ cont'd

reduced variability and shallow decelerations are more likely to be of hypoxic origin and may denote **'chronic or long-standing hypoxia'**. Clinical suspicion should increase in the presence of thick meconium-stained liquor, reduced fetal movements, IUGR, post-term, signs of infection or bleeding. In cases with adverse neonatal outcomes, it would be useful to submit the placenta and the cord for histological examination

to assess whether infection or an unhealthy placenta might have been contributory.

Fetuses with hypoxia may have a normal baseline rate, but with no accelerations, silent pattern (baseline variability below 5) and shallow decelerations (amplitude <15 beats) (see Fig. 8.3). Such a fetus may not stand the stress of labour and may die within 1 to 2 h of admission. Figure 8.6A–D shows an admission test trace with a baseline rate of 140 bpm. With the progress of labour, the baseline variability is further reduced (<5 beats) without a rise in the baseline rate and the fetus dies in a span of 40 min. There appears to be some difficulty in identifying the correct baseline rate and some may consider the baseline to be 120 bpm with accelerations. But accelerations are an abrupt increase in the heart rate and not a gradual rise whilst decelerations can be abrupt as in variable decelerations or gradual decline as in early head compression decelerations or as in late placental insufficiency decelerations. Careful attention to reducing baseline variability would also indicate that the correct baseline rate was 140 bpm with decelerations.

PLANNING MANAGEMENT

An admission test is helpful when planning the subsequent care in labour. High-risk women or women with suspicious or abnormal admission tests should have continuous EFM throughout labour. A normal admission test is an insurance policy that permits us to encourage mobilization with no further need to perform EFM for 3–4 h or until signs of the late first stage of labour are apparent. Even in the second stage of labour, a few minutes' strip of EFM after a contraction should be enough in the low-risk woman. Alternative delivery positions, the use of water immersion

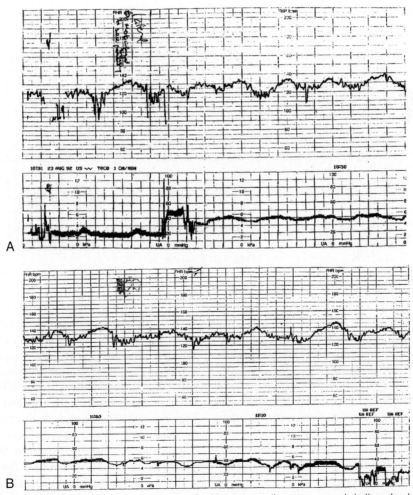

Fig. 8.6 ■ (A–D) A non-reactive trace with normal baseline fetal heart rate, silent pattern and shallow decelerations. Sudden fetal demise within 50 min of admission.

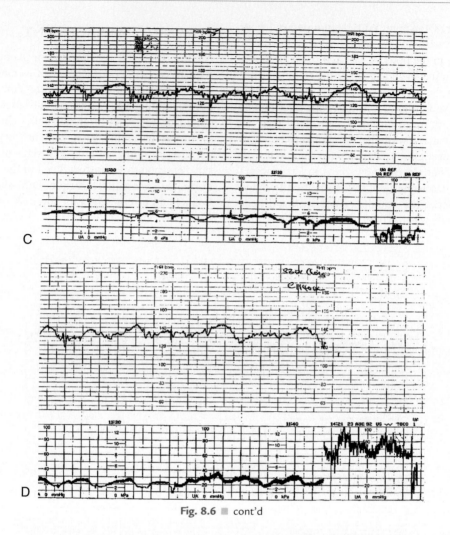

Fig. 8.6 ■ cont'd

in labour and preparations for a water birth may be more confidently pursued.

An AT followed by monitoring in the late first stage and second stage, the time of greatest stress, appears appropriate.

How Long Should an Admission Test Last?

An AT should last as long as necessary until it is normal. This implies a consideration of fetal sleep and fetal behavioural states. If two accelerations, a normal rate and normal variability are seen in the first 5 min then that is very reassuring. It is useful if two or more contractions are witnessed with no decelerations during this time as this will provide reassurance that there is no stress to the fetus with the contractions. If EFM is commenced at the start of a quiescent phase for the fetus then it will need to be continued until the fetus reawakens but one can be reassured to continue observation in the absence of decelerations with contractions. Most ATs should last 15 to 30 min; however, the mother with a normal trace in 5 min, keen for mobilization and natural labour, should not be monitored unduly. Midwives can gain more confidence in the home-birth situation by applying these principles and using a hand-held Doptone, especially with the graphic display of the FHR trace. There is no contraction recording with Doppler devices and hence the need to palpate the contractions and start listening toward the end and after the contraction to detect any decelerations.

The parents should be given a choice, as in every matter; however, the choice provider may find it difficult to offer truly informed choices. It seems to us the simple question that the parents should be asked is 'Would you like us to check that your baby is OK?'

EFM should be appropriate: not too much, not too little. Advances in technology have made it possible to use simple devices to provide the same information as with larger more complicated machines.

REFERENCES

[1] National Institute for Health and Care Excellence (NICE). Intrapartum care for healthy women and their babies. NICE Clinical Guideline 3 December 2014;190. Online. Available at: https://www.nice.org.uk/guidance/cg190/resources/intrapartum-care-for-healthy-women-and-babies-35109866447557 [accessed 10.08.16].

[2] Birthplace in England Collaborative Group. Perinatal and maternal outcomes by planned place of birth for healthy women with low risk pregnancies: the Birthplace in England national prospective cohort study. BMJ 2011;343:d7400.

[3] Hobel CJ, Hyvarinen MA, Okada DM, et al. Prenatal and intrapartum high risk screening. 1. Prediction of the high risk neonate. Am J Obstet Gynecol 1973;117(1):1–9.

[4] Arulkumaran S, Gibb DMF, Ratnam SS. Experience with a selective intrapartum fetal monitoring policy. Singapore J Obstet Gynecol 1983;14:47–51.

[5] Ingemarsson I, Arulkumaran S, Ingemarsson E, et al. Admission test: a screening test for fetal distress in labour. Obstet Gynecol 1986;68:800–6.

[6] Fleischer A, Schulman H, Jagani N, et al. The development of fetal acidosis in the presence of an abnormal fetal heart rate tracing. I. The average for gestation age fetus. Am J Obstet Gynecol 1982;144(1):55–60.

[7] Bix E, Reiner LM, Klovning A, et al. Prognostic value of the labour admission test and its effectiveness compared with auscultation only: a systematic review. Br J Obstet Gynaecol 2005;112:1595–604.

[8] Mires G, Williams F, Howie P. Randomised controlled trial of cardiotocography versus Doppler auscultation of fetal heart at admission in labour in low risk obstetric population. BMJ 2001;322:1435–98.

[9] Impey L, Reynolds M, MacQuillan K, et al. Admission cardiotocography: a randomised controlled trial. Lancet 2003;361(9356):465–70.

[10] Malcus P, Gudmundson S, Marsal K, et al. Umbilical artery Doppler velocimetry as a labour admission test. Obstet Gynecol 1991;77:10–6.

[11] Sarno APJ, Ahn MO, Brar H, et al. Intrapartum Doppler velocimetry, amniotic fluid volume and fetal heart rate as predictors of subsequent fetal distress. Am J Obstet Gynecol 1989;161:1508–11.

[12] Chamberlain PF, Manning FA, Morrison I, et al. Ultrasound evaluation of amniotic fluid. I. The relationship of marginal and decreased amniotic fluid volumes to perinatal outcome. Am J Obstet Gynecol 1984;150(3):245–9.

[13] Crowley P, O'Herlihy C, Boylon P. The value of ultrasound measurement of amniotic fluid volume on the management of prolonged pregnancies. Br J Obstet Gynaecol 1984;91:444–5.

[14] Chauchan SP, Washburne JF, Magann EF, et al. A randomized study to assess the efficacy of the amniotic fluid index as a fetal admission test. Obstet Gynecol 1995;86:9–13.

[15] Teoh TG, Gleeson RP, Darling MR. Measurement of amniotic fluid volume in early labour is a useful admission test. Br J Obstet Gynaecol 1992;99:859–60.

[16] Chua S, Arulkumaran S, Kurup A, et al. Search for the most predictive tests of fetal well-being in early labour. J Perinat Med 1996;24:199–206.

[17] Phelan JP, Ahn MO, Smith CV, et al. Amniotic fluid index measurements during pregnancy. J Reprod Med 1987;32:601–4.

[18] Chan FY, Lam C, Lam YH, et al. Umbilical artery Doppler velocimetry compared with fetal heart rate monitoring as a labor admission test. Eur J Obstet Gynecol Reprod Biol 1994;54:1–6.

[19] Keegan KAJ, Waffarn F, Quilligan EJ. Obstetric characteristics and fetal heart rate patterns of infants who convulse during the newborn period. Am J Obstet Gynecol 1985;153:732–7.

[20] Van der Merwe P, Gerretsen G, Visser G. Fixed heart rate pattern after intrauterine accidental decerebration. Obstet Gynecol 1985;65:125–7.

[21] Menticoglou SM, Manning FA, Harman CR, et al. Severe fetal brain injury without evident intrapartum trauma. Obstet Gynecol 1989;74:457–61.

[22] Schields JR, Schifrin BS. Perinatal antecedents of cerebral palsy. Obstet Gynecol 1988;71:899–905.

[23] Leveno KJ, William ML, De Palma RT, et al. Perinatal outcome in the absence of antepartum fetal heart rate accelerations. Obstet Gynecol 1983;61:347–55.

[24] Devoe LD, McKenzie J, Searle NS, et al. Clinical sequelae of the extended non-stress test. Am J Obstet Gynecol 1985;151:1074–8.

[25] Brown R, Patrick J. The non-stress test: how long is long enough? Am J Obstet Gynecol 1981;141:646–51.

[26] Phelan JP, Ahn MO. Perinatal observations in forty-eight neurologically impaired term infants. Am J Obstet Gynecol 1994;171:424–31.

[27] Herbst A, Ingemarsson I. Intermittent versus continuous electronic fetal monitoring in labour. Br J Obstet Gynaecol 1994;101:663–8.

9 ASSESSMENT OF UTERINE CONTRACTIONS

DONALD GIBB ■ SABARATNAM ARULKUMARAN

Effective contractions of the uterus are an essential prerequisite for labour and vaginal delivery. The progress of labour, evidenced by dilatation of the uterine cervix and descent of the presenting part, is the final result of contractions. During the journey through the birth canal the fetus is intermittently squeezed and stressed by the contractions. Maternal blood flow into the uteroplacental space ceases when the intrauterine pressure (IUP) exceeds the pressure of flow of blood into the retroplacental area. A well-grown fetus with good placental reserve tolerates this as 'normal stress' and displays no change or minimal benign change in the fetal heart rate (FHR). A compromised fetus may show cardiotocograph (CTG) changes with this stress. Reduction of the retroplacental pool of blood due to contractions will be manifested as late decelerations. In a normal fetus, stress can be brought about by cord compression, which will be shown as variable decelerations. The presence of atypical variable decelerations indicates that there is cord compression and at the same time there is reduction of the retroplacental pool of blood (e.g., atypical variable decelerations with late recovery, or a combination of variable and late decelerations; that is, the onset of deceleration coincides with the onset of the contraction but the recovery of the FHR to baseline is after the offset of the contraction).

CONTRACTION ASSESSMENT

The standard method of assessing contractions is with the hand placed on the abdominal wall over the anterior part of the uterine fundus. This permits observation of the duration and frequency of contractions.

A subjective impression is gained of their strength. This is entirely adequate if performed intermittently in normal low-risk labour. The pattern of contractions present is very variable. They are often present, although infrequent, before labour begins. A simple assessment of the frequency of contractions (number per 10 minutes [min]), the mean duration (in seconds [s]) and a subjective impression of strength (weak, moderate or strong) usually suffices. The method of recording this is seen on the partogram (see Fig. 2.3).

Continuous monitoring of uterine contractions is performed using external tocography. The tocograph transducer (Fig. 9.1A) is a strain gauge device detecting forward movement and change in the abdominal wall contour due to change in shape of the uterus with an anterior thrust on account of the contraction; it records continuously what the hand feels intermittently. The transducer is placed without the application of jelly on the anterior abdominal wall, near the uterine fundus, and secured with an elastic belt. It is important to adjust the tension of the belt for comfort and to secure an adequate recording. Currently tocograph transducers are available that are kept in position with an adhesive instead of a belt, avoiding the restriction of a belt. These transducers are also cordless, thus allowing the mother to move freely. The recent intervention is to have optical sensors in the toco transducer to detect maternal pulse rate and record it on the CTG allowing the observer to distinguish maternal heart rate from that of an FHR (see Fig. 9.1B and C).

Obesity and a restless mother can compromise uterine contraction recording; in these circumstances, and in other clinical situations, there may be a role for IUP

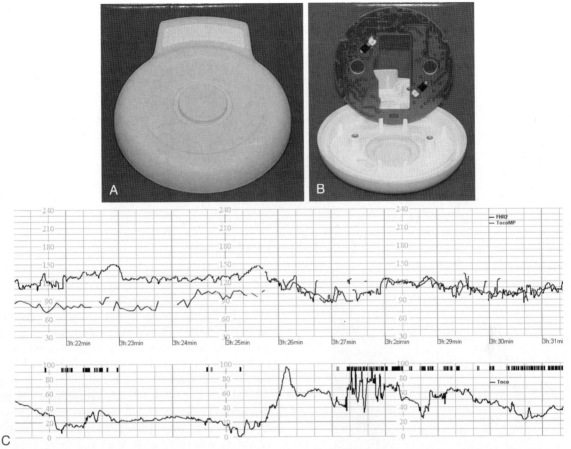

Fig. 9.1 ■ (A) An external toco transducer showing a central button that is connected to a pressure sensor gauge which perceives the contractions with the change of the abdominal contour during contractions. (B) Toco transducer that has two optical sensors that help to record maternal pulse continuously. (C) The recording shows continuous recording of the maternal pulse on the cardiotocograph, obtained from the two optical sensors in the toco transducer (B). (Courtesy – Philips Ltd.)

measurement using an intrauterine catheter (Fig. 9.2). Figure 9.3 shows a transducer-tipped catheter which obviates the need for fluid-filled catheters. IUP measurement is the most effective method of recording contractions. Figure 9.4 shows the change in recording in an obese mother seen after converting from external to internal tocography over a period of 20 min. IUP measurement is the most effective method of recording contractions.[1–5]

CLINICAL APPLICATION

What are the indications for continuous tocography? In general, continuous external tocography is performed when continuous FHR monitoring is being performed. This is a pragmatic, practical approach; however, it ignores the rationale that the indication for each is separate although they may be related. If the FHR pattern is normal and the labour progress is normal then continuous tocography does not provide additional useful information, and the woman could be spared the discomfort of the tocography belt. There remains the issue that if the fetal heart pattern or labour progress becomes abnormal then information is already available about the pre-existing contractions, which are of importance. Hence, two-channel monitoring as seen on the recording paper – of the heart rate and the contractions – is standard. Whenever the

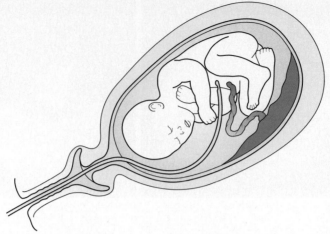

Fig. 9.2 ■ An intrauterine catheter in situ.

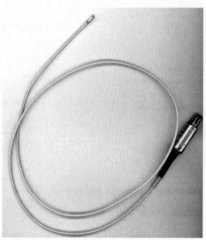

Fig. 9.3 ■ Transducer-tipped intrauterine catheter with the sensor in the recessed area.

heart rate is abnormal or labour progress is abnormal requiring treatment, the need for continuous contraction observation is clear.

Figure 9.5 shows an admission test performed on a woman with tightenings. Although the tocographic tracing suggests frequent regular contractions, the woman was not experiencing pain and did not go into labour that day. The tocography transducer may detect localized contractions that are not propagating throughout the uterus, as also shown with marked irregularity in Figure 9.6.

The Diagnosis of Labour Is Not Made From the Cardiotocograph

What are the indications for internal tocography using an IUP catheter? Other than in an obese or restless mother, external tocography provides enough information to interpret an abnormal fetal heart tracing. The management of the contractions observed depends on the frequency of contractions, whether there are FHR changes and the observed progress of labour. If induction of labour or augmentation of slow labour is non-progressive then the more complete information derived from an IUP catheter might be useful.[6] However, available data suggest that, in most of these situations, titration of the oxytocin infusion rate based on frequency and duration of contractions recorded by external tocography is adequate.[7,8] The exception might be the obese, restless mother or the nullipara with an occipitoposterior position with poor progress of labour requiring a high-dose infusion of oxytocin.

Poor labour progress in a woman with a previous caesarean section scar, there is the concern for the integrity of the uterine scar. Scar rupture or dehiscence may not manifest scar pain, tenderness, vaginal bleeding or alteration in maternal pulse and blood pressure, or may manifest these some time after the event; FHR or uterine activity changes may be an earlier sign of scar disruption.[9,10] In some centres there is a link between the indication for internal FHR monitoring with an electrode and internal pressure monitoring

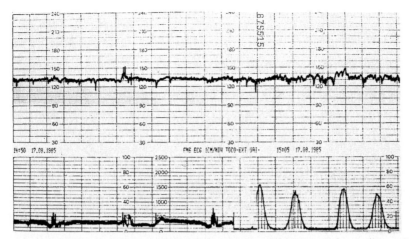

Fig. 9.4 ■ Change in recording of the uterine contractions when converted from external recording to intrauterine pressure recording.

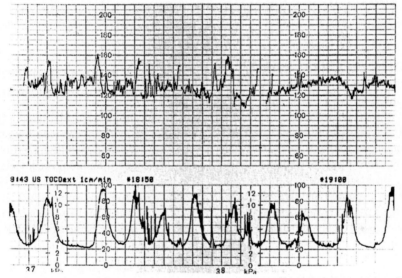

Fig. 9.5 ■ Recording of uterine contractions by external topography but mother did not experience painful contractions.

with a pressure catheter. There is no logic in this as each addresses separate issues.

The last decade has seen a shift away from the technological imperative that use of machines must be good. Sensitive care with good human relations should be the core of what we do. Excessive use of internal monitoring is invasive psychologically as well as physically. High-quality modern electronic monitors allow us to record the baby's heart without recourse to a fetal scalp electrode.

An IUP catheter is even more invasive. There are cases of infections, placental bleeds and uterine perforations associated with catheter use. At the same time there are no randomized trials showing benefits

of such technology. There may be exceptional cases where they are useful, but they should only be used by medical professionals who are familiar with them and trained in their use. There may be centres where their use is permitted for research under controlled conditions including ethical approval.

CONTRACTION MONITORING WITH THE USE OF PROSTAGLANDINS FOR INDUCTION OF LABOUR

It is important to record uterine contractions and the FHR prior to, and soon after, insertion of vaginal

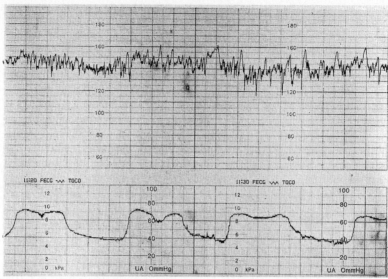

Fig. 9.6 ■ Marked irregularity of uterine contractions observed by external tocography which does not influence management.

prostaglandin (PG) pessaries or gels. The rate of absorption of PG varies from woman to woman based on the pH, temperature and moisture content of the vagina and whether there is infection, inflammation or abrasion in the vagina. Rapid absorption can give rise to tetanic or too-frequent contractions, which need not be painful but may cause suspicious/abnormal FHR changes, including prolonged deceleration that may compromise the fetus if prompt action is not taken. Action can be in the form of removing the PG pessary if possible and/or use of tocolytic agents to abolish uterine contractions.

CONTRACTION MONITORING AFTER EXTERNAL CEPHALIC VERSION

A small abruption leading to uterine irritability and FHR changes may occur following external cephalic version (ECV) without much pain, and hence the need to monitor uterine contractions and the FHR for 30–60 min after ECV. If uterine irritability is observed with too-frequent contractions (five in 10 min), the FHR may become abnormal and hence the recording should be continued until no, or infrequent, uterine contractions are observed and the FHR pattern is normal.

CONTRACTION MONITORING IN CASES OF SUSPECTED ABRUPTION

In the presence of clinical features suggestive of abruption (i.e., bleeding and/or continuous abdominal pain if there is uterine irritability), uterine contractions and the FHR should be monitored. Consideration should be given for early delivery if the FHR trace is unsatisfactory with uterine irritability, if fetal maturity is not a major concern. In the presence of uterine irritability and suspicious or pathological FHR pattern, the FHR can suddenly deteriorate leading to the need for an emergency delivery.

In-Coordinate Uterine Contractions

Abnormalities of contraction shape, frequency and tone are seen as polysystole (merging of contractions), paired contractions and tachysystole (more than five contractions in 10 min) and hypertonia (increase in baseline pressure). In-coordinate uterine contractions can be associated with normal labour and are not an indication for oxytocin unless they are inefficient in producing the expected cervical dilatation. The use of oxytocin in dysfunctional labours may improve the efficiency but may also increase the in-coordinate nature of uterine contractions.

Polysystole

Polysystole refers to contraction frequency greater than six in two consequent 10-min periods. They may appear as a single contraction with more than one peak and the tone in between the peaks not falling to the baseline. Paired contractions have a relaxation time of less than 60 s in between successive contractions. Contractions which merge to form a sustained contraction lasting for greater than 3 min are defined as tetanic contractions. They are not generally seen in natural labour and are due to use of oxytocin infusion. When contractions do not merge but the baseline pressure is elevated by more than 20 mmHg for more than 3 min, they are called hypertonic contractions (see Fig. 10.2). Tetanic contractions will cut off perfusion to the retroplacental pool of blood, while hypertonic activity will reduce perfusion. Spiral arterioles are completely compressed with an IUP of 30 mmHg. IUP reaches up to 60 mmHg in normal labour, with relaxation in between to replenish the intervillous space. Sustained elevation of the baseline tone causes compromise to uteroplacental perfusion and fetal oxygenation.

REFERENCES

1. Arulkumaran S, Yang M, Chia YT, et al. Reliability of intrauterine pressure measurements. Obstet Gynecol 1991;78:800–2.
2. Caldeyro-Barcia R, Sica-Blanco Y, Poseiro JJ, et al. A quantitative study of the action of synthetic oxytocin on the pregnant human uterus. J Pharmacol Exp Ther 1957;121(1):18–31.
3. Hon EH, Paul RH. Quantitation of uterine activity. Obstet Gynecol 1973;42:368–70.
4. Steer PJ. The measurement and control of uterine contractions. In: Beard RW, editor. The current status of fetal heart rate monitoring and ultrasound in obstetrics. London: Royal College of Obstetricians and Gynaecologists; 1977. p. 48–68.
5. Gibb DMF. Measurement of uterine activity in labour – clinical aspects. Br J Obstet Gynaecol 1993;110:28–31.
6. Arulkumaran S, Gibb DMF, Ratnam SS, et al. Total uterine activity in induced labour – an index of cervical and pelvic tissue resistance. Br J Obstet Gynaecol 1985;92:693–7.
7. Arulkumaran S, Chua S, Chua TM, et al. Uterine activity in dysfunctional labour and target uterine activity to be aimed with oxytocin titration. Asia-Oceania J Obstet Gynaecol 1991;17:101–6.
8. Chua S, Kurup A, Arulkumaran S, et al. Augmentation of labor: does internal tocography produce better obstetric outcome than external tocography? Obstet Gynecol 1990;76:164–7.
9. Beckley S, Gee H, Newton JR. Scar rupture in labour after previous lower segment caesarean section: the role of uterine activity measurement. Br J Obstet Gynaecol 1991;98:265–9.
10. Arulkumaran S, Chua S, Ratnam SS. Symptoms and signs with scar rupture: value of uterine activity measurements. Aust N Z J Obstet Gynaecol 1992;32:208–12.
11. Gibb DMF, Arulkumaran S. Assessment of uterine activity. In: Whittle M, editor. Clinics in obstetrics and gynaecology. London: Baillière Tindall; 1987. p. 111–30.

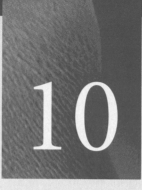

THE USE OF OXYTOCIN AND FHR CHANGES

DONALD GIBB ■ SABARATNAM ARULKUMARAN

Oxytocin is commonly used for induction and augmentation of labour. Many medico-legal cases relate to the misuse of oxytocin. Oxytocin does not have a direct influence on the fetal heart rate (FHR) or on the controlling cardiac centres in the brain, as is the case with some anaesthetic and antihypertensive drugs. Its influence is indirect via increased uterine activity, mostly due to increased frequency of contractions or baseline pressure (hypertonus). Increase in duration or amplitude of contractions can also lead to FHR changes. There is confusion on terminology of uterine contractions. Abnormal contractions may be tachysystole due to hyperstimulation with the use of Syntocinon or hypertonus when there is a rise of the intrauterine baseline pressure. Tachysystole or hyperstimulation refers to contractions in excess of 5 in 10 minutes (min).

Figure 10.1 shows fetal bradycardia due to 'tetanic' or sustained contractions lasting for 3–4 min, caused by oxytocin hyperstimulation. Because the fetus was healthy with a normal reactive FHR prior to the episode, the transient bradycardia returned to normal once the oxytocin infusion was reduced and the abnormal contractions ceased.

Figure 10.2 shows fetal bradycardia due to 'hypertonic' uterine activity. The baseline pressure was elevated by 15 mmHg for 3 min despite regular contractions. The raised baseline pressure reduced the perfusion in the retroplacental area, leading to FHR changes, which returned to normal once the baseline pressure settled to normal levels, restoring normal perfusion.

Figure 10.3 shows a reactive trace with one contraction in 3 min. An oxytocin infusion was commenced 10 min from the start of this segment at a rate of 1 mU/min. This resulted in the late decelerations and changes seen in the latter part of the trace. The contraction recording shows no increase in frequency or duration of contractions, nor an increase in baseline pressure, but does show an increase in amplitude of contractions. Discontinuation of the infusion resulted in return of the FHR trace to normal.

The FHR changes associated with oxytocin infusion may be caused by compression of the cord with contractions, or by the reduction in placental perfusion due to increased intrauterine basal pressure and frequent contractions cutting off the blood supply to the placenta. Pressure on the head or supraorbital region of the fetus can also give rise to variable decelerations due to vagal stimulation. The rate of increasing hypoxia due to cord compression or reduction of retro-placental perfusion would be shown by a deteriorating trend of the FHR – rise in baseline rate, increase in depth and duration of decelerations, reduction in inter-deceleration intervals and finally baseline variability. The rate of decline of pH depends on the FHR pattern observed and the physiological reserve of the fetus.[3] A rapid decline would be anticipated in post-term and growth-restricted fetuses and those with reduced amniotic fluid with thick meconium, infection or intrapartum bleeding. Fortunately, in the vast majority of patients who are given oxytocin, FHR changes of a worrying nature are not encountered and most changes, even when they occur, are transient and

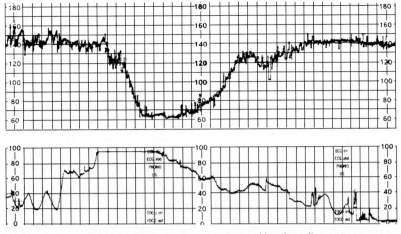

Fig. 10.1 ■ Sustained contraction and bradycardia.

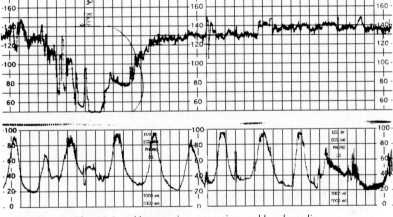

Fig. 10.2 ■ Hypertonic contraction and bradycardia.

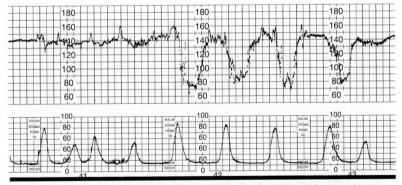

Fig. 10.3 ■ Normal trace and subsequent decelerations with oxytocin.

resolve spontaneously, or with reduction of the dose or transient cessation of the infusion. It is good practice to run a strip of cardiotocograph (CTG) prior to commencing oxytocin to make sure of good fetal health as reflected by a normal reactive FHR pattern; *if the trace is pathological then oxytocin should not be used*, as it can cause further hypoxia to the fetus by reducing the perfusion to the placenta by additional contractions.

If a pathological FHR pattern is observed in a woman on an oxytocin infusion, the infusion should be stopped, or its rate reduced, and the woman nursed on her side to improve the maternal venous return, and thus her cardiac output, in order to increase the uteroplacental perfusion. Oxygen inhalation by the mother and an intravenous bolus of tocolytic drugs to abolish uterine contractions are given in some centres. Such practice may not be necessary in the majority of cases and its value in other cases is debatable. It is known that oxytocin becomes bound to receptors, and for its action to be reduced to half can take up to 45 min after stopping the oxytocin infusion. A case may be made for the use of a bolus dose of a tocolytic drug in a patient with a grossly abnormal (pathological) FHR pattern.[4,5] There is little merit in performing a fetal scalp blood pH measurement in a patient receiving oxytocin as the FHR changes are iatrogenic. If the test is done soon after a prolonged bradycardia, or after ominous decelerations, it may show acidosis, prompting the performance of an emergency caesarean section (see Fig. 10.4A). On the other hand, if a fetal blood sample (FBS) is not taken and time is allowed, the FHR recovers and within 30–40 min the scalp blood pH is likely to be normal (see Fig. 10.4B). On many occasions, there is no need to measure scalp blood pH and the oxytocin infusion can be restarted after the return of the FHR to normal.

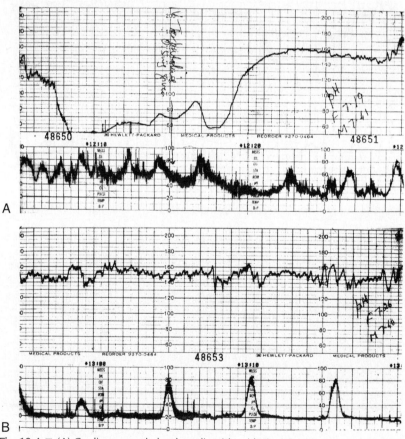

Fig. 10.4 ▪ (A) Cardiotocograph: bradycardia with acidosis; (B) reversion to normal pH.

It is debatable for how long the oxytocin infusion should be stopped once the FHR abnormality is detected. It is usual to wait until the abnormal features disappear and the reactive trace is seen; however, it is known that, although the trace returns to normal, the fetal blood biochemistry reflected on scalp blood testing may still show a low pH, high PCO_2 and low PO_2. Additional time is required for the blood biochemistry to become normal, which takes place rapidly once the FHR is normal. Noting the time necessary for the FHR to become normal after the oxytocin infusion is stopped, and allowing an equal length of time to elapse before restarting the infusion, would allow the biochemistry to become normal. Doubling the time period in this way before restarting oxytocin should cause little or no FHR changes compared with restarting oxytocin immediately after the FHR returns to normal. It is also advisable to resume the infusion at half the previous dose rate to reduce the chances of hyperstimulation or abnormal FHR changes. As the sensitivity of the uterus to oxytocin increases with the progress of labour,[6] such careful titration is likely to produce fewer problems of abnormal FHR changes or uterine hyperstimulation. Increased uterine activity in the late first stage and second stage of labour may be due to reflex release of oxytocin due to distension of the cervix and the upper vagina (i.e., the Ferguson reflex).[7]

Figure 10.5A shows abnormal FHR changes produced by oxytocic hyperstimulation. Even with immediate cessation of oxytocin infusion it takes about 45 min for the FHR to return to normal (see Fig. 10.5B) and hence sufficient time should be given for recovery. Although it is advisable to stop the oxytocin infusion as soon as abnormal FHR patterns, such as decelerations or bradycardia, are observed, it may be adequate to reduce the oxytocin dose by half or less when the FHR is normal but there is abnormal uterine activity.

Figure 10.6A shows a reactive FHR at the beginning, but decelerations and tachycardia subsequently develop owing to increased frequency of contractions. In Figure 10.6B the FHR becomes tachycardic; towards the latter part of the trace, the dose of oxytocin was reduced to half and the tocographic transducer was adjusted. In Figure 10.6C the contractions have become less frequent, the FHR has settled to a normal baseline rate and is followed by a reactive pattern.

In cases of failure to progress in labour, oxytocin is commenced to augment uterine contractions. This may bring about FHR changes when the dose is increased to achieve the optimal target frequency of contractions. If the dose is reduced, the FHR pattern returns to normal but the uterine activity drops to suboptimal levels with no progress in labour. When FHR changes are encountered in such a situation, they may be transient and it may be worth stopping and restarting oxytocin or reducing the dose. However, if pathological FHR changes appear when oxytocin is recommenced despite these efforts, it may be better to deliver abdominally. In selected cases, further time may be given to see whether the labour will progress without the use of oxytocin. An alternative would be to stop oxytocin and perform a fetal blood sample 20–30 min later and, if the pH is normal, to restart the oxytocin infusion and observe for progressive rise in the baseline rate, increase in depth and duration of decelerations, shortening of inter-deceleration intervals and reduction of baseline variability. In the absence of these changes a cervical assessment can be made to assess progress after 2–4 hours (h). If there is no progress then caesarean section may be appropriate. If there is adequate progress a repeat pH can be performed. The rate of decline of pH related to the rate of progress of cervical dilatation can be deduced and a decision made to allow progress if the pH is unlikely to be acidotic by the time of anticipated delivery. Obviously the plans need to be changed if there is a worsening FHR pattern.

With experience and confidence in interpretation of CTG, performance of FBS may not be necessary. One should note the cervical dilatation at the time of commencement of oxytocin. Continuous CTG monitoring helps to observe FHR changes. If there are decelerations and tachycardia and if there is reduction in baseline variability, or if the decelerations are lasting longer than the duration of the FHR at the baseline in between decelerations, then oxytocin infusion should be stopped and cervical dilatation assessed. If there is acceptable progress, one could wait for the FHR pattern to return to near normal (back to the pre-oxytocin baseline rate) with more time at the baseline in between decelerations, then the oxytocin infusion could be restarted and progress assessed in a couple of hours. If the CTG becomes abnormal the whole clinical situation should be reassessed and a decision

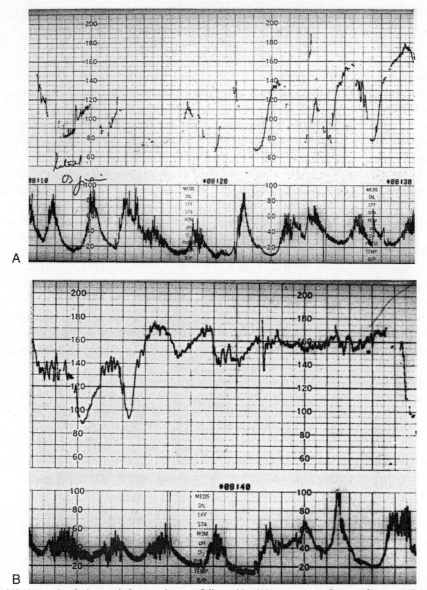

Fig. 10.5 ■ (A) Hyperstimulation and abnormal trace, followed by (B) correction of trace after cessation of oxytocin.

made. If there is no or very slow progress at the time abnormal CTG was observed, one should consider stopping the oxytocin infusion and progressing to a caesarean section or resorting to FBS if one still wants to continue with oxytocin infusion. The stopping and starting of oxytocin may cause the labour to be a little longer but the baby should be born in good condition.

In induced labour, in the absence of disproportion, the uterus has to perform a certain amount of uterine activity depending on the parity and cervical score to achieve vaginal delivery. Considering this, it may be possible to achieve optimal uterine activity that does not cause FHR changes but is adequate to bring about slow but progressive cervical dilatation.[8] The labour may be a little longer, during which time adequate contractions are generated to achieve vaginal delivery. However, such management needs intrauterine catheters and equipment to compute uterine activity, and

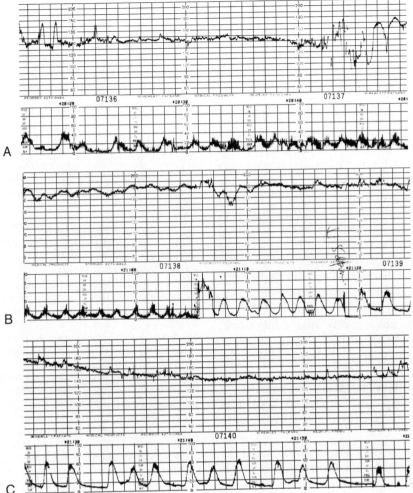

Fig. 10.6 ■ (A) Increased frequency of contractions: changes in trace; (B) sustained tachycardia; (C) reversion to normal after reduction of oxytocin.

it may not be always possible to achieve optimal uterine activity without FHR changes and achieve vaginal delivery.

MEDICO-LEGAL CONSIDERATIONS

Oláh and Steer have reviewed the use and abuse of oxytocin.[2] They highlight that, although recognizing the appropriate use of oxytocin may be helpful, its abuse is implicated in many cases with adverse outcomes and medico-legal sequelae.

The major concerns with oxytocin and medico-legal issues relate to the following:

- inadequate uterine contraction monitoring;
- poor technical quality of the FHR trace;
- cessation of monitoring the FHR or uterine contractions much earlier than the time of delivery;
- commencement of oxytocin when there are major risk factors (e.g., thick meconium-stained scanty fluid, evidence of chorioamnionitis and a suspicious or pathological FHR trace);
- failure to recognize that the uterus is contracting greater than five in 10 min despite no increase in oxytocin infusion and failure to reduce or stop the oxytocin infusion, thereby

causing a pathological FHR pattern such as prolonged decelerations and fetal compromise;

■ failure to use tocolytics in some cases to alleviate the problem early, as time is needed for oxytocin-induced contractions to reduce/abate;

■ failure to recognize that prolonged decelerations following a normal FHR trace may recover, but the trace may not recover despite stopping oxytocin if the FHR prior to the decelerations was suspicious or abnormal;

■ when prolonged decelerations occur the fetal monitor may record the 'maternal heart rate', which may not be recognized by the caregiver;

■ the fetus may be affected with hypoxia despite prompt action (e.g., delivery), but the caregiver may be liable if the prolonged FHR decelerations were caused by uterine hyperstimulation;

■ oxytocin should be used with caution when there are FHR changes as it may make things worse; careful consideration should be given to deliver rather than to augment or induce labour;

■ in the presence of thick meconium and scanty fluid, meconium aspiration syndrome is a possibility with late or atypical prolonged decelerations suggestive of hypoxia even without acidosis;

■ decelerations in early labour, or prolonged decelerations with the use of oxytocin may imply impending scar rupture with oxytocin in a woman with a previous scar;

■ if the FHR shows what appears to be accelerations, they may be decelerations if the baseline rate does not settle and show an 'active and quiet sleep cyclicity' pattern with continuation of the recording for 2 h.

REFERENCES

[1] Inducing labour. NICE guideline [NG207]. Published: 04 November 2021. Available at: https://www.nice.org.uk/guidance/ng207. [Accessed 08 January 2022].

[2] Oláh KSJ, Steer PJ. The use and abuse of oxytocin. TOG 2015;17(4):267.

[3] Arulkumaran S, Ingemarsson I. Appropriate technology in intrapartum fetal surveillance. In: Studd JWW, editor. Progress in obstetrics and gynaecology. Edinburgh: Churchill Livingstone; 1990. p. 127–40.

[4] Ingemarsson I, Arulkumaran S, Ratnam SS. Single injection of terbutaline in term labor. I. Effect on fetal pH in cases with prolonged bradycardia. Am J Obstet Gynecol 1985;153(8):859–65.

[5] Ingemarsson I, Arulkumaran S, Ratnam SS. Single injection of terbutaline in term labor. II. Effect on uterine activity. Am J Obstet Gynecol 1985;153(8):865–9.

[6] Sica BY, Sala NL. Oxytocin. In: Caldeyro-Barcia R, Heller H, editors. Proceedings of an international symposium. London: Oxford: Pergamon Press; 1961. p. 127–36.

[7] Ferguson JKW. A study of the motility of the intact uterus at term. Surg Gynecol Obstet 1941;73:359–66.

[8] Arulkumaran S, Gibb DMF, Ratnam SS, et al. Total uterine activity in induced labour – an index of cervical and pelvic tissue resistance. Br J Obstet Gynaecol 1985;92(7):693–7.

11

MECONIUM, INFECTION, ANAEMIA AND BLEEDING

LEONIE PENNA

INCREASING FETAL RISK

This chapter reviews some specific clinical circumstances that increase the risk that the fetus will develop intrauterine hypoxia with a risk of adverse neonatal outcome. This association means that extra vigilance is needed in observing any abnormalities seen on the cardiotocograph (CTG) and that a change in context for recommending intervention is sometimes needed.

MECONIUM

The passage of meconium is common, resulting in meconium-stained amniotic fluid (MSAF) in about 10% (range 7%–22%) of term deliveries.[1] Most meconium is physiological and is due to spontaneous peristaltic contraction of the bowel which may occur with fetal maturity without an adverse event as part of normal fetal behaviour. The incidence of MSAF at 42 weeks is about 30% and this is less as gestational age and thus physiological maturity reduces.[1] In preterm gestations, meconium is uncommon (<5% at 34 weeks).[2] There is a strong association with fetal infection, particularly listeriosis, in these circumstances. There is also an increased incidence of MSAF reported in pregnancies complicated by obstetric cholestasis, gastroschisis and fetal bowel pathologies.[3] This may reflect fetal vomiting or regurgitation.

Why Is Meconium Important to Neonatal Outcome?

- Meconium is an independent risk factor for poor neonatal outcome, with an increased risk of cerebral palsy (CP) in neonates where meconium was observed during labour.[4]
- Meconium passage can occur as a result of hypoxic stress; reduction in oxygen results in an adrenergic response with redistribution of blood to essential organs and reduction in blood supply to non-essential organs including the bowel. Peristaltic bowel contractions and relaxation of the anal sphincter are adrenergic responses that can result in the passage of meconium.
- Meconium is acidic and if it enters the fetal lungs it causes a chemical pneumonitis and respiratory distress in a condition called meconium aspiration syndrome (MAS). Pulmonary hypertension can occur as a complication of this condition.[5]
- Meconium can enter the fetal lungs if the fetus makes reflex gasping movements, which are known to occur in response to sudden acute hypoxia or as an end stage in slow-developing subacute hypoxia.[6]
- Overall about 5% of infants born following a labour complicated by MSAF will develop MAS. Physiological meconium can result in MAS if a hypoxic event occurs causing the fetus to gasp, but the risk is greater with thicker meconium. MAS is a serious condition causing significant morbidity and mortality (accounting for about 2% of all perinatal mortality in the UK in 2007).[7]
- Thick meconium is known to increase the risk of cord spasm in utero with resultant increased risk of hypoxaemia and hypoxia.[8]

- Meconium inhibits the phagocytic activity of macrophages in amniotic fluid (AF) and may enhance bacterial growth, increasing the risk that intrauterine infection will occur. It has been suggested that the fetal systemic inflammation that occurs in chorioamnionitis may be an important factor in why fetuses develop MAS.[9]

Meconium and Fetal Monitoring

Although most meconium is physiological, its association with adverse neonatal outcome means that it must be considered as a potential complication of labour, with a review of risk factors in the pregnancy and labour. The relationship of meconium to fetal infection is important and often overlooked and this should be considered if the fetal heart pattern becomes abnormal.

Historically meconium has been graded as follows:

- grade 1 – light meconium with good volumes of AF
- grade 2 – heavier meconium staining but still with a good volume of AF
- grade 3 – very heavy meconium with reduced AF.

As these descriptions are highly subjective, more recent classifications suggest the use of just two categories:[10]

LIGHT = meconium contamination where there is a large volume of AF.

- Light meconium will usually have occurred some time prior to rupture of membranes and be present at the time of spontaneous rupture of membranes or of amniotomy. Light meconium is likely to be physiological but the possibility of hypoxaemic stress and of infection should still be considered in all cases.
- If the woman is at low risk for the development of infection or hypoxia, then intermittent auscultation (IA) can be recommended. In women planning birth outside an obstetric unit (home birth or midwifery-led unit), this plan should be carefully scrutinized with consideration of transfer to the obstetric unit.[10]
- In a woman with risk factors or where the clinic circumstances suggest it is less likely to be physiological (gestations below 38 weeks), CTG monitoring should be recommended.[10]

- If IA suggests any possible fetal heart rate (FHR) abnormality, including a rising baseline rate (even if within normal limits), then conversion to CTG monitoring should be recommended.[10]

HEAVY = meconium contamination where there is reduced AF resulting in the meconium being much more concentrated.

- Although heavy meconium may be present at the time of rupture of membranes, it more commonly develops during labour. Heavy meconium, in small volumes of fluid, is much less likely to be physiological and has a much higher association with MAS,[11] and thus careful review is needed of all maternal risk factors.
- CTG monitoring should be recommended in all cases.[7]

Other Management Decisions

In cases of pre-labour rupture of membranes (>34 weeks), meconium is an indication for recommending immediate induction of labour. This is as much because of the increased risk of infection associated with meconium as the more commonly cited concerns about fetal well-being.[12]

If the CTG trace is normal (see Ch. 6) then no additional action needs to be taken even in the presence of very thick meconium. Although meconium is a cofactor for the development of infection, there is no good evidence that the administration of antibiotic to otherwise-asymptomatic women improves fetal outcome and so is not recommended[13] – although the most recent Cochrane review on the subject concluded that antibiotics may reduce chorioamnionitis and recommended further research in this area.[14] Likewise, studies of amnioinfusion in labours complicated by thick meconium have not shown any benefits for the neonate and so this is not recommended.[15]

If the CTG trace becomes suspicious, then the possibility of hypoxaemic stress must be considered. The decisions about management must be individualized but will depend on parity, stage and progress in labour and the wishes of the parents according to their view of the risks involved. As MSAF is associated with a 1-in-20 risk of MAS, it is essential that women and their partners are included in decision-making where options for management exist. The normal intrauterine resuscitation measures of maternal repositioning, intravenous (IV) fluids, reduction in oxytocin dose and IV antibiotics (if infection is suspected) should be undertaken without delay.

If the CTG trace becomes pathological, the risk of fetal gasping and MAS increases.[11] This is particularly so if prolonged decelerations occur. The combination of thick meconium, clinical signs of infection and a pathological CTG is particularly ominous and immediate delivery is indicated.

There is a common perception that fetal blood sampling (FBS) should not be performed in the presence of heavy meconium and a pathological trace because there is a high risk that fetal hypoxia is developing and thus a fear of MAS. The threshold for FBS is definitely altered, with delivery preferable in many cases. However, not to do FBS in all circumstances incurs maternal risk related to emergency caesarean section and so decisions should be individualized. FBS for a pathological trace with meconium prior to potentially difficult instrumental delivery and in women with a high expectation of vaginal delivery in the near future are examples of situations where FBS may be the appropriate management.

Not all fetuses with subacute hypoxia will pass meconium, and fetuses that experience a sudden severe hypoxic event such as uterine rupture may also not pass meconium. Also, even if present, new meconium may not be seen with a deeply engaged head as occurs in the second stage of labour. Therefore, the absence of Meconium stained liquor in the presence of an abnormal FHR pattern should not be considered as reassuring.

Clear AF is reassuring. Thick, fresh meconium in a situation of high risk is of great concern.

An attempt should be made in all cases with a fetal heart trace not classified as normal to release AF from above the presenting part if necessary; this is done by pushing the presenting part gently upward. If no fluid appears, then the possibility of oligohydramnios and potential fetal compromise must be considered.

INFECTION

Maternal infection is common during labour, with 1%–4% of labours complicated by chorioamnionitis.[16] Infection is an important cofactor in the development of hypoxia as evidence shows that infection increases the risk of poor neonatal outcome.

Why Is Infection Important to Neonatal Outcome?

- Clinical (and sub-clinical based on histology of the placenta) chorioamnionitis during labour is an independent risk factor for poor neonatal outcomes including CP.[17] Microbial toxins or cytokines released during maternal infection can cause 'fetal inflammatory response syndrome' (FIRS) with fetal cytokine production. FIRS has been implicated as a cause of cystic periventricular leucomalacia and CP without evidence of direct infection in the fetus.[18]
- Clinical chorioamnionitis can result in a neonatal infection with pneumonia, meningitis or generalized sepsis. Fetal infection in utero may cause fetal tachycardia (the mother having a normal pulse), with a resultant increase in basal metabolic rate (BMR) with increased oxygen/energy requirements for normal functions and the risk of a more rapid decompensation than would occur in the non-infected fetus if hypoxia developed.
- Maternal infection causes a shift of the oxygen dissociation curve to the right due to hyperthermia reducing oxygen delivery to the fetus, which results in greater hypoxaemia and a higher risk of developing hypoxia.[19]

Maternal pyrexia from any cause will increase the fetal temperature owing to a reduction in passive heat loss. Maternal pyrexia can cause concomitant fetal tachycardia. Even in the absence of fetal infection, pyrexia and tachycardia will increase both the fetal BMR and the fetal energy requirements (in adults an increase in BMR of up to 13% per degree rise in temperature[20]). This increases the chances that the hypoxaemia occurring from intermittent cord compression is more likely to result in the development of hypoxia. This can occur in the healthy fetus, but there is an even greater risk for a fetus already compensating for a stress such as placental insufficiency.

Infection and Fetal Monitoring

The fact that fetal neurological injury may occur secondary to infection, and that infection per se may reduce the threshold for hypoxia and for hypoxic brain injury, means that CTG monitoring could avoid superimposing intrapartum hypoxia on intrauterine infection. For these reasons, continuous electronic fetal monitoring is recommended in any labour where there is a significant risk of infection.[10,21]

Although this is a standard recommendation, the effect of chorioamnionitis on FHR patterns is uncertain as no pattern specific to chorioamnionitis alone has ever been identified. The most common finding is fetal tachycardia due to fetal sepsis or as a response to pyrogens crossing the placenta from the mother. Reduced variability and variable-type decelerations have been reported in a number of small case series but have not been proven to have any specific association with infection.[22]

Term fetuses with both intrauterine infection and non-reassuring FHR patterns are at a higher risk of developing CP than fetuses with only one risk factor,[23] suggesting that if evidence of hypoxia develops in the presence of infection then swift intervention is required.

There is often concern that the use of FBS in the presence of infection carries a risk of inoculating the fetus with infection, that capillary stasis from sepsis could give erroneous results and that the association of infection with CP means that any suspicion of hypoxia requires immediate delivery, which are cited as reasons for not doing it. However, there is no evidence to confirm these concerns, which remain theoretical.

Adopting a 'no FBS' policy in suspected chorioamnionitis will result in unnecessary caesareans, both in women who do not actually have infection and in those with infection where the CTG has been falsely suggestive of hypoxia, and there is no evidence that caesarean section will alter the outcome for the neonate but it may be associated with increased infective morbidity in the mother.[24]

Fetuses with infection who develop hypoxaemia will potentially deteriorate more rapidly, developing severe hypoxia and asphyxia; therefore in deciding whether to undertake FBS the presence of other risk factors for the development of hypoxia, slow progress or the development of fetal heart abnormalities in early labour (especially in a primigravida) mitigate against performing this test. If there are no other risk factors for hypoxia and labour is established and progressing well then prompt FBS can be considered. Evidence suggests that FBS is not a quick procedure[25] and in the presence of infection it should be undertaken by the most experienced clinician available and abandoned (with recourse

to caesarean) if a sample is not obtained in a timely manner. If the CTG abnormality persists after a normal FBS result, an early repeat test (30 minutes [min] or less) should be undertaken owing to the risk of more rapid deterioration in chorioamnionitis, and caesarean section is recommended if there has been any significant deterioration in the pH or base excess.

Other Management Decisions

Other infections can cause direct effects on the fetal heart with resultant changes in the CTG. These include infections by organisms such as cytomegalovirus (CMV) and *Listeria*;[26] no specific pattern has been described but, for an abnormal CTG with no other obvious explanation, these diagnoses should be considered, especially if a history of recent non-specific febrile illness or other risk factors for infection is elicited. Apparently unprovoked reduced variability, decelerations and a tachycardia without other explanation may be seen on fetal monitoring.

In severe maternal sepsis, a maternal metabolic acidosis may develop as part of the disease process. Even in the absence of fetal infection or maternal hypotension, an uncorrected maternal acidosis will result in a slowly developing fetal acidosis due to the inability of the placenta to clear hydrogen ions and lactate.[27] The trace may show reduction in variability and unprovoked decelerations without the development of tachycardia (Fig. 11.1). Correction of the maternal condition may reverse the fetal condition, but this needs to be done as quickly as possible to avoid the risk of long-term neurological damage due to lactic acidosis. At viable gestations where the maternal condition is considered sufficiently stable, delivery by emergency caesarean section should be considered (Fig. 11.2).

FETAL ANAEMIA

There are many reasons why a fetus can develop anaemia in pregnancy (Table 11.1) but all are rare.

Occasionally, the risk can be anticipated from the maternal history, but in the majority of cases, anaemia occurs in an unheralded fashion either because risk factors have gone undetected or because the anaemia occurs from an unpredictable event. As untreated fetal anaemia can result in fetal death or survival with neurological damage it is essential that all clinicians are familiar with FHR patterns that may indicate anaemia.

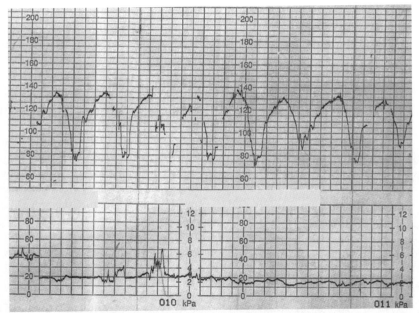

Fig. 11.1 ■ 37 weeks: severe maternal metabolic acidosis secondary to peritonitis from a ruptured appendix. Prompt emergency caesarean section (and appendicectomy) with good maternal and neonatal outcome.

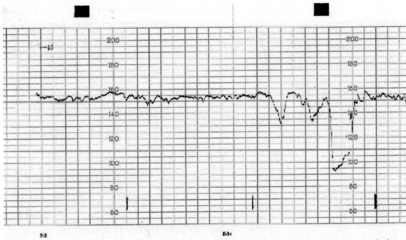

Fig. 11.2 ■ 34 weeks: recent travel to the USA presented with reduced fetal movements. Ultrasound showed mild ascites. Delivery was by caesarean section with poor condition at birth. Investigations confirmed fetal/neonatal *Listeria* infection. There was normal neurodevelopment at age 5 years.

Why Is Anaemia Important to Neonatal Outcome?

- Anaemia reduces the oxygen-carrying capacity of the fetal blood, making hypoxaemia more likely.
- Haemoglobin and plasma bicarbonate are the major buffers utilized by the fetus to neutralize hydrogen ions and maintain extracellular pH within a critical range, avoiding effects in the CNS and cardiovascular system. Any reduction in haemoglobin will reduce the fetal ability to withstand even short periods of anaerobic metabolism and this worsens with the degree of anaemia.
- A fetus with chronic anaemia compensates for the low haemoglobin by a hyperdynamic circulation,

but as the anaemia progresses this will result in cardiac failure and fetal hydrops.[28]

■ A fetus with sudden blood loss is in 'double jeopardy': firstly of becoming hypovolaemic due to loss of circulating blood volume and secondly of losing buffering ability that allows the fetus to withstand minor hypoxic events.

TABLE 11.1
Causes of Fetal Anaemia

Acute Anaemia (Hypovolaemic)	Chronic Anaemia (Normovolaemic)
Any acute fetomaternal haemorrhage, e.g., placental abruption, abdominal trauma	Fetal infections, e.g., CMV, parvovirus
Bleeding from vasa praevia	Alloimmune haemolytic anaemia, e.g., rhesus or other red cell antibodies
Transplacental delivery (CS) for placenta praevia	Genetic syndromes, e.g., Blackfan–Diamond anaemia, aneuploidy
Acute TTTS in monochorionic twins	Chronic TTTS in monochorionic twins

CMV, Cytomegalovirus; *CS,* caesarean section; *TTTS,* twin-to-twin transfusion syndrome.

■ FHR changes occur only when severe anaemia is present, and thus prompt action is required following a suspicion of anaemia to ensure a good outcome.

Anaemia and Fetal Monitoring

A sinusoidal pattern of the fetal heart in severe fetal anaemia was first described in 1972 and is now accepted as pathognomonic of fetal anaemia[29] if it is a persistent feature on monitoring. The pathophysiology underlying the pattern remains enigmatic, but two factors are changes in the autonomic nervous activity secondary to hypoxia from the reduced oxygen-carrying capacity and baroreceptor-mediated changes due to hypovolaemia.

The sinusoidal pattern is not seen in fetuses with mild anaemia and occurs only when the haemoglobin is below 100 g/l.[30]

■ There are two distinct types of sinusoidal patterns; both exhibit reduced variability: *Typical sinusoidal* is the pattern associated with chronic anaemia (e.g., rhesus disease) where there is no reduction in the circulating blood volume but a low haemoglobin. In the absence of any additional hypoxic stress, the FHR will be in the normal range and will show frequent

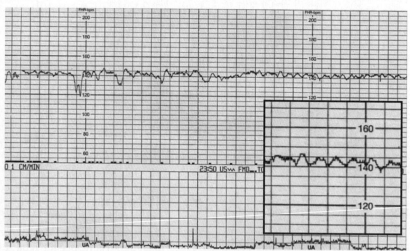

Fig. 11.3 ■ 32 weeks: admitted with reduced fetal movements. The trace shows a typical sinusoidal pattern in a fetus with parvovirus infection; note the enlarged portion of trace, which demonstrates the profound reduced variability with 'castle-wall' effect. Intrauterine transfusion was performed with good neonatal outcome.

low-amplitude (5–10 bpm) oscillations at a frequency of 3–5 per min (Fig. 11.3).

- *Atypical sinusoidal* is the pattern seen in acute anaemia where the fetus is hypovolaemic and anaemic owing to loss of circulating blood volume. The FHR will be tachycardic and show more frequent high-amplitude oscillations (15–20 bpm) with some similarity to saltatory pattern variability (Fig. 11.4).

Many CTG traces will show short periods of sinusoidal-type pattern but, as a true sinusoidal pattern does not self-correct because fetal anaemia is never transient (it takes time to recover even if the cause of the problem has resolved), these short periods interspersed with a normal trace are not significant and therefore not a cause for concern or intervention.

A pseudosinusoidal pattern describes a pattern that may be seen in non-anaemic fetuses; the pattern is not persistent and has been attributed to fetal thumb sucking and is a finding in the premature fetus. Maternal opiate use can also cause CTG changes that can be mistaken for a sinusoidal pattern.

Other Management Decisions

A fetus with significant anaemia is already coping with stress due to a reduced ability to carry oxygen and any additional stress reducing fetal gas transfer, such as normal contractions, may result in decompensation and rapid development of hypoxia. Therefore, the treatment of a persistent sinusoidal trace in labour is immediate delivery by caesarean section with availability of facilities for advanced neonatal resuscitation. Vasa praevia is a rare condition where unprotected fetal blood vessels are present in the membranes overlying the cervix, with the risk of disruption and haemorrhage when the membranes rupture.[31] Neonatal mortality rates of up to 60% are described, but prompt recognition of the significance of the atypical sinusoidal pattern associated with relatively small amounts of bleeding followed by urgent delivery will improve the outcome (Fig. 11.5).

Sinusoidal traces (usually typical pattern) may also be seen in women presenting with reduced fetal movements who are not in labour. In the absence of a history of bleeding an urgent fetal medicine opinion should be requested. Measurement of the middle cerebral artery (MCA) Doppler in the fetus will allow confirmation of fetal anaemia as the peak systolic velocity (PSV) will be elevated.[28] Steroids should be recommended in pre-term gestations and a Kleihauer–Betke test performed to look for fetomaternal haemorrhage. Treatment should be individualized depending on the suspected cause.

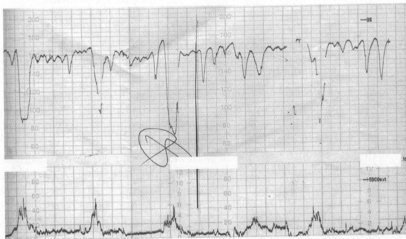

Fig. 11.4 ■ 39 weeks: admitted with contractions and light vaginal bleeding after spontaneous rupture of membranes. The trace shows an atypical sinusoidal pattern (note the raised baseline). The trace appearances were mistaken for infection until terminal decompensation. There was emergency caesarean section delivery of the neonate in very poor condition and haemoglobin 30 g/l, and early neonatal death.

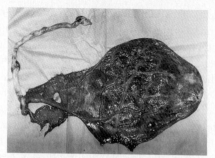

Fig. 11.5 ■ Placenta from the fetus in Figure 11.4. Membranous cord insertion and bleeding fetal vessel in an undiagnosed vasa praevia were clearly visible on examination.

MATERNAL BLEEDING

Vaginal bleeding during pregnancy is common (3%–5% of pregnancies) and may occur antenatally or as an intrapartum complication.[32]

Why Is Bleeding Important to Neonatal Outcome?

- Any antepartum haemorrhage (APH) is a risk to the well-being of the fetus as placental abruption is the cause of the bleeding in a significant number of cases.
- If abruption occurs there is separation of some part of the placental mass from the uterine wall; this may be small marginal-type abruption with no immediate fetal effect, or separation of a large area of the placenta resulting in severe fetal compromise. Separation of any part of the placenta reduces the placental area available for transfer of oxygen and nutrients to the fetus. Although the fetus is able to withstand reduction of placental area on a chronic basis (as in fetal growth restriction due to infarction) without immediate effect, a loss of a similar volume very suddenly is likely to cause changes in the FHR pattern as the fetus tries to adapt to the new situation. The addition of a stress such as contractions (intrapartum abruption) may result in decompensation unless the fetal reserve is unusually large. A sudden large separation of an area of the placenta will result in rapid and profound hypoxia and fetal decompensation regardless of whether other stresses on fetal well-being are present.

- In the absence of other causes, even very small APHs must be considered as possible abruption and at the point of presentation should be considered as potentially unstable; this could be the beginning of an evolving large abruption or a process of recurrent smaller haemorrhages, each reducing the available placental reserve for the fetus.
- Abruption is more common in pregnancies complicated by poor placentation[33] and therefore is more likely to occur in a fetus with a degree of compensated chronic placental insufficiency. Decompensation may occur even though the maternal symptoms are seemingly trivial (light bleeding and no pain).
- The possibility that bleeding could be of fetal origin should be considered, especially if the onset of even a relatively small amount of bleeding is associated with the onset of fetal tachycardia. In abruption there is a risk that fetomaternal haemorrhage will occur (further increasing fetal risk). A Kleihauer–Betke test should be requested in all cases of suspected abruption[31] and should be undertaken as soon as possible after the acute presentation. The laboratory often needs to be reminded that the test is required for clinical reasons and even in Rhesus (Rh)-positive women.

Bleeding and Fetal Monitoring

Continuous CTG and IV access should be recommended in all cases of significant intrapartum bleeding. In women presenting with APH antenatally, fetal monitoring should be commenced as soon as possible so as to confirm fetal well-being, as seemingly trivial revealed bleeding may be only part of a larger concealed bleed.

There are no specific FHR patterns that are pathognomonic of abruption. An acute massive separation of the placenta is one of the causes of a sudden-onset non-recovering fetal bradycardia – usually developing features of terminal pattern with loss of variability or a deep swinging saltatory variability. This requires urgent caesarean section and is a situation where the aim must be for delivery by 20 min to ensure a good fetal outcome; however, as this situation carries

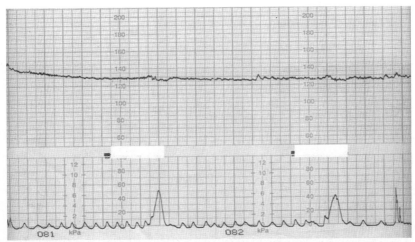

Fig. 11.6 ■ 36 weeks: admitted with significant antepartum haemorrhage in a pregnancy being monitored for pre-eclampsia. Note the reduction in variability and the contraction pattern. The cervix was very unfavourable and a decision for emergency caesarean section was made. A large retroplacental clot was present at delivery. There was a good neonatal outcome.

significant maternal risk, the need for rapid delivery must be balanced against the need for effective maternal resuscitation before surgery.

An uncomplicated tachycardia may occur as a sign of fetal stress and should be treated with maternal fluid resuscitation (essential if there is concomitant maternal tachycardia or heavy vaginal bleeding).

Late decelerations may be precipitated by intrapartum abruption as this can reduce the available placental reserve.

Persistent reduced variability in the trace in the fetus of a mother with APH should be considered as indicating impending decompensation.

If CTG abnormalities occur, then fluid resuscitation of the mother should be commenced and consideration given to delivery by urgent caesarean section (at viable gestations).

The combination of a developing fetal anaemia and compromise due to reduction in placental reserve can give rise to unusual patterns in the CTG, and so it is important that the clinician is very cautious about any CTG that is not classifiable by standard guidelines (Fig. 11.6).

Evaluation of uterine activity as shown on by the tocograph can reveal evidence of uterine irritability, which may indicate a more significant 'concealed' abruption with tracking of blood into the myometrium causing recurrent low-amplitude contractions and an increase in resting uterine tone (Fig. 11.7). These may not be palpable and the woman may not describe contractions, being more likely to describe constant pain with exacerbations. In such cases, there is a risk of sudden fetal decompensation; the management plan for care should encompass this.

Other Management Decisions

Delivery by caesarean section should be considered in all cases of non-reassuring FHRs in the presence of significant bleeding that could be due to abruption. As the rate of deterioration of the fetal condition can be rapid, FBS should not be considered.

Usually the bleeding from placenta praevia occurs following minor placental separation and therefore FHR abnormality in small bleeds is uncommon. However, in the event of a large haemorrhage, acute fetal hypoxia can occur as a result of significant separation and/or maternal hypotension. Prompt maternal fluid resuscitation is essential for both mother and fetus prior to urgent delivery by caesarean section as reversal of maternal hypotension will improve the fetal condition.[34]

Non-uterine causes of APH should not be associated with fetal compromise unless maternal hypotension occurs and thus assessment of the fetal heart is an essential clinical sign that should be recorded in relation to all vaginal bleeding.

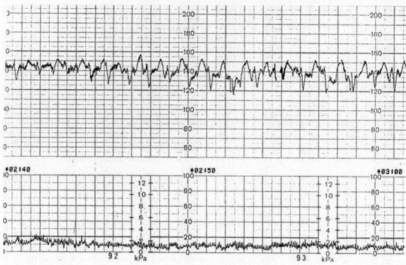

Fig. 11.7 ■ 38 weeks: admitted with a small vaginal bleed, contractions and abdominal pain. Cervix was 3 cm dilated. Note the activity on the tocograph and the cardiotocograph pattern that is difficult to classify by any normal guideline; 60 minutes later a sudden bradycardia commenced, immediate caesarean section was performed with delivery of a fresh stillborn infant. A large concealed abruption was present.

REFERENCES

[1] Cleary GM, Wiswell TE. Meconium-stained amniotic fluid and the meconium aspiration syndrome. An update. Pediatr Clin N Am 1998;45:511–29.

[2] Tybulewicz AT, Clegg SK, Fonfe GJ, et al. Preterm meconium staining of the amniotic fluid: associated findings and risk of adverse clinical outcome. Arch Dis Child Fetal Neonatal Ed 2004;89:F328–30.

[3] Collins S, Arulkumaran S, Hayes K, et al. Oxford handbook of obstetrics and gynaecology. In: Oxford medical handbooks. 3rd ed. Oxford: Oxford University Press; 2013.

[4] Berkus MD, Langer O, Samueloff A, et al. Meconium-stained amniotic fluid: increased risk for adverse neonatal outcome. Obstet Gynaecol 1994;84(1):115–20.

[5] Nair J, Lakshminrusimha S. Update on PPHN: mechanism and treatment. Semin Perinatol 2014;38(2):78–91.

[6] Guntheroth W, Kawabori I. Hypoxic apnoea and gasping. J Clin Invest 1975;56:1371–7.

[7] National Institute for Health and Clinical Excellence (NICE). Intrapartum care: care of healthy women and their babies during childbirth. NICE guideline CG55. London: NICE; September 2007.

[8] Naeye R. Can meconium in the amniotic fluid injure the fetal brain? Obstet Gynecol 1995;86:720–4.

[9] Lee J, Romero R, Lee K, et al. Meconium aspiration syndrome: a role for fetal systemic inflammation. AJOG 2016;214(3):366–e1–9.

[10] National Institute for Health and Care Excellence (NICE). Intrapartum care for healthy women and their babies. NICE clinical guideline 190 3 December 2014. Online.

Available: https://www.nice.org.uk/guidance/cg190/resources/intrapartum-care-for-healthy-women-and-babies-35109866447557 [accessed 10.08.16].

[11] Starks GC. Correlation of meconium-stained amniotic fluid, early intrapartum fetal pH, and Apgar scores as predictors of perinatal outcome. Obstet Gynecol 1980;56:604–9.

[12] Seaward P, Hannah M, Myhr T, et al. International multicentre term prelabour rupture of membranes study: evaluation of predictors of clinical chorioamnionitis and postpartum fever with prelabour rupture of membranes at term. Am J Obstet Gynecol 1997;177(5):1024–9.

[13] Shivananda S, Murthy P, Shah PS. Antibiotics for neonates born through meconium stained amniotic fluid. Cochrane Database Syst Rev 2006;4:CD006183.

[14] Sirriwachirachi T, Sangomkamhang U, Lumbiganon P, et al. Antibiotics for meconium-strained amniotic fluid in labour for preventing maternal and neonatal sepsis. Cochrane Database Syst Rev 2014;11:CD007772.

[15] Hofmeyr GJ, Xu H, Eke AC. Amnioinfusion for meconium stained liquor in labour. Cochrane Database Syst Rev 2014;1:CD000014. https://doi.org/10.1002/14651858. CD000014.pub4.

[16] Gibbs RS, Duff P. Progress in pathogenesis and management of clinical intra-amniotic infection. Am J Obstet Gynecol 1991;164:1317.

[17] Wu Y, Colford J. Chorioamnionitis as a risk factor for cerebral palsy. A meta-analysis. JAMA 2000;284(11):1417–24.

[18] Bashiri A, Burstein E, Mazor M. Cerebral palsy and fetal inflammatory response syndrome: a review. J Perinat Med 2006;34(1):5–12.

[19] White AC. The bicarbonate reserve and the dissociation curve of oxyhemoglobin in febrile conditions. J Exp Med 1925;41(3):315–26.

[20] Hardy JD, Dubois F. Regulation of heat loss from the human body. Proc Natl Acad Sci USA 1937;23(12):624–31.

[21] Ayres-de-Campos D, Spong C, Chandraharan E, FIGO Intrapartum Fetal Monitoring Expert Consensus Panel. FIGO consensus guidelines on intrapartum fetal monitoring: cardiotocography. Int J Obstet Gynecol 2015;131(1):13–24. Online. Available: https://obgyn.onlinelibrary.wiley.com/doi/full/10.1016/j.ijgo.2015.06.020. [accessed 25.11.2022].

[22] Aina-Mumuney AJ, Althaus JE, Henderson JL, et al. Intrapartum electronic fetal monitoring and the identification of systemic fetal inflammation. J Reprod Med 2007;52(9):762–8.

[23] Nelson K. Infection in pregnancy and cerebral palsy. Dev Med Child Neurol 2009;51(4):253–4.

[24] Rouse DJ, Landon M, Leveno KJ, et al. National Institute of child health and human development, maternal-fetal medicine units network. The maternal-fetal medicine units cesarean registry: chorioamnionitis at term and its duration—relationship to outcomes. Am J Obstet Gynecol 2004;191:211–6.

[25] Tuffnell D, Haw WL, Wilkinson K. How long does a fetal scalp blood sample take? BJOG 2006;113:332–4.

[26] Hasbún J, Sepúlveda-Martínez A, Hayes T, et al. Chorioamnionitis caused by *Listeria monocytogenes*: a case report of ultrasound features of fetal infection. Fetal Diagn Ther 2013;33(4):268–71.

[27] Omo-Aghoja L. Maternal and fetal acid–base chemistry: a major determinant of perinatal outcome. Ann Med Health Sci Res 2014;4(1):8–17.

[28] Désilets V, Audibert F. SOGC clinical practice guideline: investigation and management of non-immune fetal hydrops. J Obstet Gynecol Can 2013;35(10):e1–e14.

[29] Modanlou HD, Murata Y. Sinusoidal heart rate pattern: reappraisal of its definition and clinical significance. J Obstet Gynaecol Res 2004;30(3):169–80.

[30] Kariniemi V. Fetal anaemia and heart rate pattern. J Perinat Med 1982;10:167–72.

[31] Royal College of Obstetricians and Gynaecologists (RCOG). Placenta praevia, placenta praevia accreta and vasa praevia: diagnosis and management. Green-top Guideline No. 27. 3rd ed. London: RCOG Press; 2011. Online. Available: https://www.rcog.org.uk/en/guidelines-research-services/guidelines/gtg27/. [accessed 10.08.16].

[32] Royal College of Obstetricians and Gynaecologists (RCOG). Antepartum haemorrhage. Green-Top guideline No. 63. London: RCOG Press; 2011. Online. Available: https://www.rcog.org.uk/en/guidelines-research-services/guidelines/gtg63/. [accessed 10.08.16].

[33] Kroener L, Wang ET, Pisarska MD. Predisposing factors to abnormal first trimester placentation and the impact on fetal outcomes. Semin Reprod Med 2016;34(1):27–35.

[34] Paterson-Brown S, Howell C. Managing obstetric emergencies and trauma: the MOET course manual. 3rd ed. Cambridge: Cambridge University Press; 2014.

12

CARDIOTOCOGRAPHIC INTERPRETATION – ADDITIONAL CLINICAL SCENARIOS

DONALD GIBB ■ SABARATNAM ARULKUMARAN

TWIN PREGNANCY

Perinatal mortality in multiple pregnancy is considerably higher than in singleton pregnancy, and particular risks are present during labour and delivery. It is now known that this mortality is considerably increased for monochorionic twins compared with their dichorionic counterparts. The rare monoamniotic twins should be delivered by caesarean section (CS) because of the risk of cord accidents, particularly after the delivery of the first twin. There is an increasing tendency to deliver monochorionic, diamniotic twins by CS because of the risk of acute fetomaternal transfusion. If this is not done, then very careful electronic monitoring must be undertaken. Twins are generally smaller than singletons, with more pathological growth restriction. The second twin may be at greater risk of this and the ability to electronically monitor both twins continuously is therefore important. The latest generation of fetal monitors has been specially designed to perform this function. One twin can be monitored on direct electrode with the other on ultrasound, or both can be monitored using external ultrasound. To have only one machine at a woman's bedside is a considerable advantage that should be fully exploited. The Huntleigh Sonicaid prints its own paper and therefore has the novel feature of a three-channel trace (Fig. 12.1). The Hewlett–Packard and Corometrics models have a technique of printing out both traces in the same channel but in different shades (Fig. 12.2). It is critical to follow the second twin with the ultrasound transducer; however, this may prove difficult, especially in an obese mother. Assisted

delivery is performed for the same indications as in a singleton pregnancy. A senior resident doctor must supervise the delivery of the second twin and ensure continuous electronic fetal monitoring during the interval between deliveries. Such an approach permits a more-measured, less-anxious delivery process; however, this should not be used as a justification for undue prolongation of the interval.

BREECH PRESENTATION

Babies presenting by the breech are acknowledged to be exposed to more risks than those presenting by the head. The Term Breech Trial Collaborative Group's study has resulted in most breech babies being delivered by CS.[1] This is unfortunate as women who like to deliver vaginally are now being denied the opportunity of vaginal breech birth and doctors in training no longer have the opportunity to acquire this skill, which will be necessary in an emergency delivery. In fact in the Breech trial, 10% of mothers who were to be delivered by CS were delivered vaginally.

There are several risks, but intrauterine growth restriction (IUGR) and umbilical cord compression have particular implications for fetal monitoring. The footling or flexed breech has a greater chance of cord prolapse and compression of the umbilical cord in labour. This is a classical scenario for variable decelerations due to cord compression, as outlined in Chapter 5. This is one of the reasons why such cases usually have planned CS. There is also evidence that compression of the skull above the orbits by the uterine fundus is a mechanism for variable decelerations. Figure 12.3

SONICAID Meridian 800

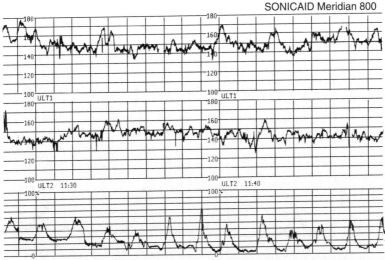

Fig. 12.1 ▪ Monitoring twins – three-channel trace (Oxford Sonicaid Meridian). (Courtesy of Huntleigh Healthcare Ltd.)

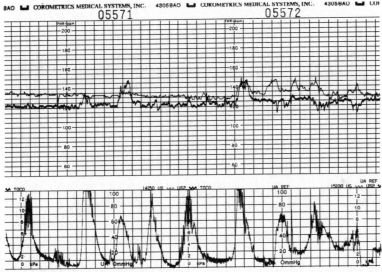

Fig. 12.2 ▪ Monitoring twins – two-channel trace (Corometrics 116). (Courtesy of GE Healthcare.)

shows a typical pattern of cord compression in a breech. Should the misfortune of umbilical cord prolapse occur then the dramatic decelerative pattern shown in Figure 12.4 may be seen. The presence or absence of developing asphyxial features, such as changes in the baseline rate, baseline variability and magnitude of the decelerations related to the speed of the evolving labour process, will relate to the outcome. Breech presentation presents special risks, and in view of these, there is little or no place for fetal blood sampling in a breech labour. The blood is more difficult to obtain from the tissues of the breech and it may be different from that obtained from scalp skin. Having understood the normal mechanisms of cardiotocography (CTG) changes in a breech, if there is a good indication for pH measurement then there is a good indication for CS.

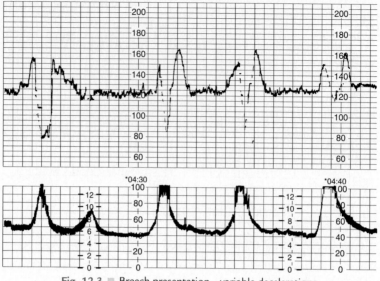

Fig. 12.3 ■ Breech presentation – variable decelerations.

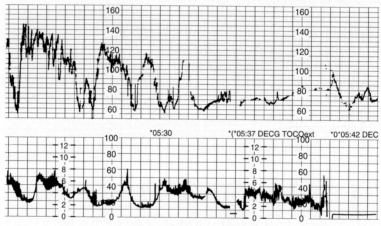

Fig. 12.4 ■ Breech cord prolapse.

BROW PRESENTATION

Brow presentation in labour in late pregnancy is very unfavourable for vaginal delivery. The mentovertical diameter, which is usually about 13 cm, presents at the pelvic brim. This leads to head compression due to a mechanical misfit. Early and variable decelerations (Fig. 12.5) are associated with this.

There are no typical features associated with a face presentation. The placement of a fetal electrode should be avoided in a recognized face presentation.

PREVIOUS CAESAREAN SECTION: TRIAL OF LABOUR WITH A SCAR

The stability of the placental circulation and utero-placental perfusion is dependent on the integrity of the uterus and its vasculature. With the dehiscence or rupture of the scar, the major uterine blood vessels may become stretched and torn, compromising the perfusion of the placenta (see Fig. 13.4A and B). There is also the possibility of the umbilical cord prolapsing through the dehisced scar, giving rise to

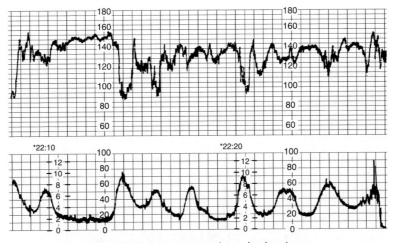

Fig. 12.5 ■ Brow presentation – decelerations.

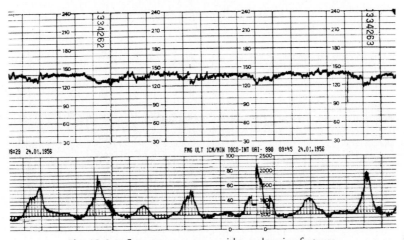

Fig. 12.6 ■ Scar rupture – trace with no alarming features.

a dramatic cord compression pattern (see Fig. 14.1A–F). It is, therefore, believed that changes in the fetal heart rate (FHR) as a result of this may be one of the first signs of 'scar dehiscence' where the myometrium has dehisced but the peritoneum is intact or 'scar rupture' where the myometrium and peritoneum have dehisced. The other signs of scar dehiscence/rupture, such as scar pain, tenderness, vaginal bleeding or alterations in maternal haemodynamics, are notoriously late and unreliable. Figure 12.6 shows a trace from a woman having a trial of scar where, at laparotomy shortly after the trace, the scar was found to have ruptured. Figure 12.7 shows another trial of labour where emergency CS was undertaken for prolonged

bradycardia with a suspicion of scar dehiscence. The baby was delivered by immediate CS (<15 minutes [min] from the decision to delivery), and had Apgar scores of 4 at 1 min improving to 7 at 5 min, making a good recovery. There were no signs of placental abruption, scar dehiscence or any other explanation for the abnormal tracing. Figure 12.8 illustrates another case where the fetus was already passing into the peritoneal cavity with a relatively normal trace and subsequently good outcome. Presumably, there was some maintenance of placental perfusion. Continuous electronic FHR monitoring in a trial labour with a scar may be helpful in the diagnosis of scar dehiscence/rupture, although this is variable.

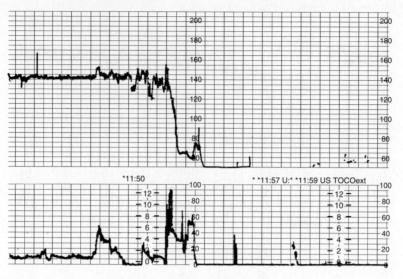

Fig. 12.7 ■ Prolonged bradycardia.

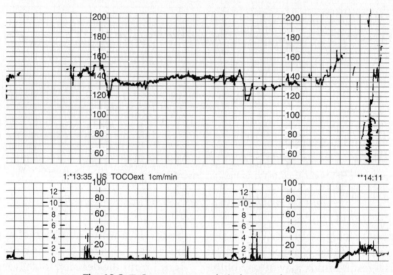

Fig. 12.8 ■ Scar rupture – relatively normal trace.

SEVERE HYPERTENSION

Women suffering from severe hypertensive disease of pregnancy have at least two possible reasons for having an abnormal CTG. The first is the disease itself and its possible association with IUGR; the second is medication. Antihypertensive drugs, by their very nature, have effects on the maternal and fetal cardiovascular systems. Methyldopa leads to reduction in baseline variability and accelerations. Beta-blocking drugs result in reduced baseline variability and accelerations.[2] Figure 12.9 shows the trace of a fetus whose mother was being treated with labetalol for her hypertension; in spite of numerous fetal movements, accelerations are limited and baseline variability reduced. The picture is confounded by medication in these high-risk pregnancies, and complementary tests such as biophysical profile and Doppler studies are appropriate.

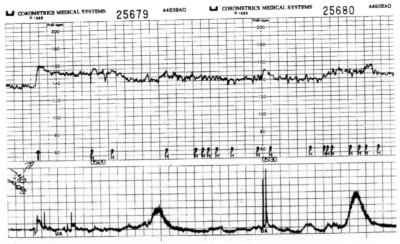

Fig. 12.9 ■ Hypertension treated with beta-blocker.

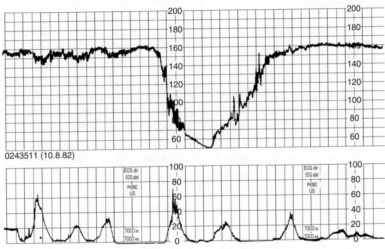

Fig. 12.10 ■ Deceleration – eclamptic fit.

ECLAMPSIA

A convulsion represents a major stress to the fetus, which it may not survive. It is likely that such a fetus is already suffering from IUGR because of severe pre-eclampsia. Figure 12.10 shows a trace during an eclamptic fit. After any major acute stress, it is important to check fetal condition by ultrasound scan or Doppler transducer of CTG before CS.

The mother's condition must be stabilized before she faces the further challenge of caesarean delivery. If the fetal heart tracing is not of major concern after the convulsion, then assessment and preparation for 1–2 hours (h) is reasonable. Undue haste may lead to maternal complications.

MEDICATION

High-risk women may be on multiple drug therapy. Figure 12.11 shows a trace from a woman with a functioning transplanted kidney who had been prescribed azathioprine, ciclosporin, prednisolone, antibiotics and atenolol. The low baseline is remarkable.

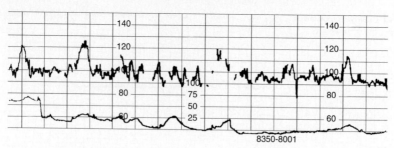

8350-8001

Fig. 12.11 ■ Unusual trace – multiple drug therapy.

Other tests of fetal well-being were normal. The trace remained normal in induced labour and the baby was in excellent condition at birth.

A baseline rate below 100 beats per min (bpm) in a non-hypoxic fetus is exceptional.

EPIDURAL ANAESTHESIA

The insertion of an anaesthetic agent into the epidural space can be associated with a degree of instability of the maternal vascular system. Provided the preceding trace has been normal then this represents a stress that the fetus can withstand. After attention is paid to the circulating volume, and vascular stability returns, then the trace returns to normal. This is a form of stress test. However, if the preceding trace has not been normal then it is wise to apply a scalp electrode before the manipulation for insertion of the epidural to facilitate monitoring. If the preceding trace has been abnormal, then a more ominous situation may develop. Figure 12.12A is a trace erroneously not recognized to be abnormal before the insertion of the epidural. The cervix was already 3 cm dilated and the trace should have prompted membrane rupture, which would have revealed thick meconium and facilitated the application of a scalp electrode. Unfortunately, the stress of epidural insertion resulted in serious asphyxial CTG changes (Fig. 12.12B) and the birth by immediate CS of a compromised baby.

SECOND STAGE OF LABOUR

The second stage is a time of very specific changes in the mechanical effects resulting from descent of the fetus. In a cephalic presentation, the initial appearances of early decelerations result from head compression. It is commonly seen in a multiparous mother in good labour. The onset of progressive early decelerations is a sign of the second stage before it has been confirmed by vaginal examination or the appearance of the head at the perineum.

Decelerations are common in the second stage.

Early decelerations gradually becoming deeper and developing variable features are characteristic of the second stage of labour. Reassurance is provided by a good recovery from each deceleration and a return to normal rate and normal variability before the next contraction (Fig. 12.13). Under these circumstances, assisted delivery is not necessary except for other reasons relating to maternal condition. Signs of evolving hypoxia are increase in depth and duration of decelerations, shortening of inter-deceleration intervals which are shorter than the duration of the decelerations, gradual tachycardia and reduced baseline variability in between and during decelerations (Fig. 12.14). Other features of concern are additional late decelerations (Fig. 12.15) and failure of FHR to return to the baseline rate after decelerations (Figs 12.16 and 12.17).[3]

Prolonged bradycardia necessitates delivery.

Failure of the FHR to return to the baseline, and especially failure to recover to at least 100 bpm, is a serious sign and delivery should be undertaken. Figure 12.16 is an example where the doctor was called within 3 min of a bradycardia. At that point the fetal heart then recovered. There was a further bradycardia of 3 min, which did not then recover. At 6 min the mother was prepared, at 9 min the forceps were prepared and at 12 min the forceps delivery was performed with the baby born in good condition.

The 3, 6, 9 and 12 min Rule

- 3 min: call the doctor
- 6 min: prepare the mother
- 9 min: prepare the forceps
- 12 min: deliver the baby

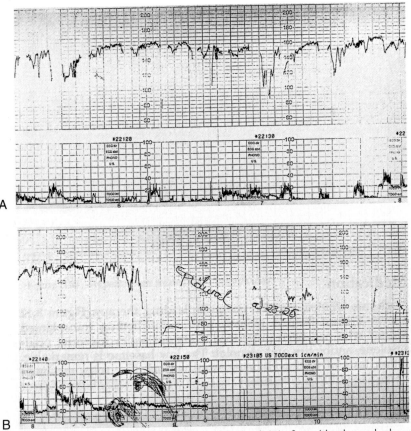

Fig. 12.12 ■ (A) Abnormal trace not recognized before insertion of epidural; (B) after epidural, grossly abnormal fetal heart rate pattern, leading to operative delivery.

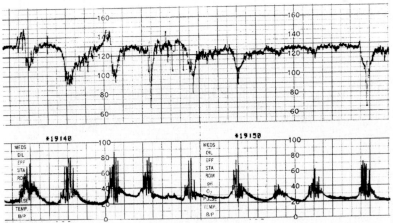

Fig. 12.13 ■ Normal second-stage fetal heart rate trace – variable decelerations.

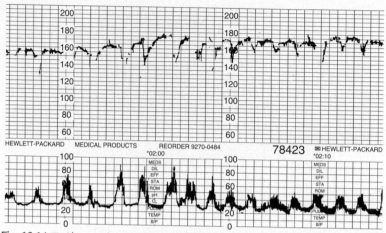

Fig. 12.14 ■ Abnormal second-stage fetal heart rate trace – developing tachycardia.

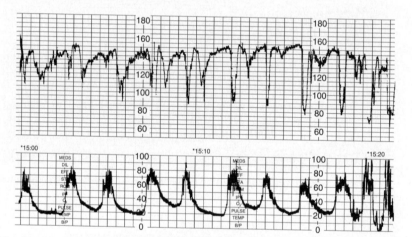

Fig. 12.15 ■ Abnormal second-stage fetal heart rate trace – additional late decelerations.

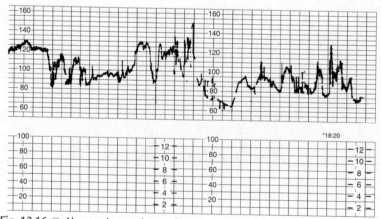

Fig. 12.16 ■ Abnormal second-stage fetal heart rate trace – prolonged bradycardia.

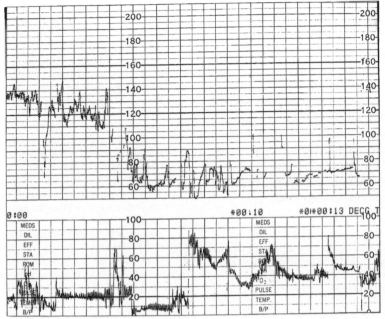

Fig. 12.17 ■ Abnormal second-stage fetal heart rate trace – prolonged bradycardia.

A delay of 20 min or more may result in an asphyxiated baby.

With a head on or near the perineum, one should try to achieve an early delivery. There is no need for washing, gowning, draping and catheterization. A pair of gloves and an instrument such as a Kiwi cup are sufficient. Time is of the essence.

PROLONGED DECELERATIONS IN THE FIRST STAGE OF LABOUR

The clinical context of the prolonged deceleration needs to be examined as to whether it is likely to be reversible (e.g., due to supine posture, following a vaginal examination, due to hypotension with administration of epidural anaesthesia, hyperstimulation due to oxytocin infusion) or irreversible (e.g., abruptio placenta, cord prolapse, scar rupture). If a reversible clinical factor is present, appropriate action should be taken. With the recovery of the deceleration, labour is allowed to continue with continued surveillance. If there is no sign of recovery by 9 min, then delivery should be carried out. A normal or suspicious FHR pattern prior to prolonged deceleration is likely to recover with corrective measures. If the prolonged deceleration is due to an irreversible factor, immediate delivery in this situation will necessitate a CS unless she reaches full dilatation and the head is below spines permitting an assisted vaginal delivery.

There are several publications in the literature that have given the audit findings of the decision-to-delivery interval, and onset of bradycardia to delivery interval.[4-7] These studies show that in a reasonable proportion of cases, delivery was possible by 20 min, and in a further considerable proportion of cases, within 30 min. The discussion is related to the possibility of such timings in a busy set-up, especially if the registrar is busy attending to another case. The recommendations of the Royal College of Obstetricians and Gynaecologists to have consultant presence in the labour ward for longer periods, especially for 24 h in units delivering more than 6000 cases, may help in such situations.[8] The aim of the teaching of 3-, 6-, 9-, 12- and 15-min guidance is to emphasize the urgency of the situation in the presence of prolonged decelerations. The greater the urgency, the lower the FHR, e.g., 50 bpm compared with 80 bpm as the perfusion per minute is much less, the longer the deceleration, absent baseline variability and in clinical situations that indicates disruption of placental perfusion such as uterine rupture and abruption. Presence of an experienced neonatal paediatrician will help in optimal resuscitation as delay or inadequate resuscitation will prolong the hypoxic insult. Rarely sudden prolonged bradycardia may occur from a suspicious trace and this may be due to infection and resuscitation of the neonate may not result in good outcome. In such cases, it would be useful to have the histology of the placenta and the umbilical cord. Histological findings of chorioamnionitis would suggest infection as the cause of poor outcome. Swabs for Group B (GpB) streptococcus from the placenta and the newborn should be performed in such cases.

REFERENCES

[1] Hannah ME, Hannah WJ, Hewson SA, et al. Planned caesarean section versus planned vaginal birth for breech presentation at term: a randomised multicentre trial. Term Breech Trial Collaborative Group. Lancet 2000;356(9239):1375–83.

[2] Montan S, Solum T, Sjöberg NO. Influence of the beta 1-adrenoceptor blocker atenolol on antenatal cardiotocography. Acta Obstet Gynecol Scand Suppl 1984;118:99–102.

[3] Melchior J, Bernard N. Second stage fetal heart rate patterns. In: Spencer JAD, editor. Fetal monitoring – physiology and techniques of antenatal and intrapartum assessment. Tunbridge Wells. Castle House Publications; 1989. p. 155–8.

[4] Bloom SL, Leveno KJ, Sponge CY, et al. Decision-to-incision times and maternal and infant outcomes. Obstet Gynecol 2006;108:6–11.

[5] Livermore LJ, Cochrane RM. Decision to delivery interval: a retrospective study of 1,000 emergency caesarean sections. J Obstet Gynaecol 2006;26(4):307–10.

[6] Tuffnel DJ, Wilkinson K, Beresford N. Interval between decision and delivery by caesarean section-are current standards achievable? Observational case series. BMJ 2001;322:1330–3.

[7] MacKenzie IZ, Cooke I. What is a reasonable time from decision-to-delivery by caesarean section? Evidence from 415 deliveries. Br J Obstet Gynaecol 2002;109:498–504.

[8] Royal College of Obstetricians and Gynaecologists (RCOG). The future role of the consultant. London: RCOG Press; 2006.

13

CARDIOTOCOGRAPHIC INTERPRETATION: MORE DIFFICULT PROBLEMS

DONALD GIBB ■ SABARATNAM ARULKUMARAN

Cardiotocography (CTG) patterns that are of specific concern are described in this chapter:

1. Prolonged deceleration (bradycardia) that can cause acute hypoxic compromise.
2. The dying fetus due to gradually developing hypoxia.
3. Chronic or pre-existing or long-standing hypoxia.
4. Pre-terminal fetal heart rate (FHR) patterns.
5. Inadvertent recording of the maternal heart rate (MHR) mimicking the FHR not being recognized by staff leading to adverse outcome.

PROLONGED DECELERATION (BRADYCARDIA)

Prolonged FHR deceleration (bradycardia) (FHR <80 beats per min [bpm]) for less than 3 minutes (min) is considered suspicious, and that for greater than 3 min is regarded as abnormal. Some literature defines prolonged deceleration as an FHR that drops to less than 100 bpm. The lower the heart rate and longer the FHR remains low the greater the chance of acidosis. A deceleration of greater than 3 min could be due to a reversible or an irreversible clinical situation. Irreversible causes of acute hypoxia due to cord compression or prolapse, abruptio placentae or scar dehiscence need to be acted upon immediately. If the prolonged deceleration is due to a reversible cause such as an epidural top-up, vaginal examination and uterine hyperstimulation, simple measures such as adjusting the maternal position, stopping the oxytocin infusion, attending to

hydration and giving oxygen by face mask may correct the condition. A patient who presents with continuous abdominal pain, vaginal bleeding, a tender, tense or irritable uterus and prolonged fetal bradycardia is likely to have suffered an abruption and warrants immediate delivery (see Ch. 11). Those in whom scar dehiscence or rupture is suspected, and those with cord prolapse, may present with prolonged bradycardia and need immediate delivery.

Most cases of prolonged bradycardia with no major pathology will show signs of recovery towards the baseline rate within 6 min. There is no place for a fetal scalp blood sample in this situation and it may make things worse.

If the clinical picture does not suggest abruption, scar dehiscence or cord prolapse, and if the fetus is appropriately grown at term with clear amniotic fluid and a reactive FHR pattern prior to the episode of bradycardia, return back to the baseline FHR pattern within 9 min is to be expected. The recovery toward the normal baseline within 6 min with good baseline variability at the time of the bradycardia and during recovery are reassuring signs, and one should wait with confidence that the FHR will revert to the normal baseline with a normal pattern. There is no place for a fetal scalp blood sample in this situation. The staff should hold their nerve with confidence. If there are no signs of recovery toward the baseline rate by 6 min, action should be taken to determine the cause, to determine cervical dilatation and to consider delivery. If the cervix is fully dilated and the head is low, a forceps or ventouse delivery should be carried out, but a caesarean section (CS) may be preferred if the cervix is not fully dilated or the head is high. This CS is considered category 1 or immediate CS in terms of the classification for the urgency with which it should be done. Category 1 should have a specific code or term assigned, such as 'code red' or 'immediate', CS, in order to mobilize all the staff (obstetricians, anaesthetists, additional midwifery staff, theatre staff, operating department assistants and paediatricians) needed to accomplish delivering the baby within 30 min of the decision being made. Obviously the decision should be made as early as possible but without overreaction. The best policy may be for the midwife and the doctor in that room to push the bed to the theatre, while the midwife on duty calls for the anaesthetist, paediatric and theatre staff. Early entry into the theatre offers the opportunity for more people to help with the various tasks of setting up an IV line, sending blood for Hb and 'group and save', catheterization and explaining to the couple the need for CS and reassuring them.

A 45-year-old multiparous woman was well known to the medical staff and midwives. A diagnosis of term labour was made at 22.00 hours (h) when the cervix was 5 cm dilated and the initial CTG was normal (Fig. 13.1A). Shortly before midnight, a prolonged bradycardia became manifest after an otherwise-normal trace (Fig. 13.1B). The midwife correctly annotated 'FHR' at the end of this strip of trace. Figure 13.1C shows the heart rate improving with good variability; however, the inexperienced obstetric registrar decided to perform a CS and consequently the trace shows 'discontinued for theatre'. Not surprisingly, the Apgar scores were 9 at 1 min and 10 at 5 min. If the trace had not been disconnected it would have reverted to normal; a premature decision led to an unnecessary CS in a multiparous woman in whom labour was probably progressing rapidly. A longer contraction duration or transient cord compression might account for the deceleration. The diagnosis was 'obstetric registrar's distress'!

If the FHR does not show signs of recovery by 9 min the likelihood of acidosis is increased, and one should take action to deliver the fetus as soon as possible.[1] The clinical picture has to be considered while anxiously awaiting the FHR to return to normal. Fetuses who are post-term, growth restricted, have no amniotic fluid or have thick meconium-stained fluid at rupture of membranes are at a greater risk of developing hypoxia.

Those with an abnormal or suspicious FHR trace prior to the episode of bradycardia are also at a greater risk of hypoxia developing within a short time. In these situations, it may be better to take action early if the FHR fails to return to normal. If uterine hyperstimulation due to oxytocics is the cause, oxytocin infusion should be stopped. Inhibition of uterine contractions with a slow bolus intravenous or subcutaneous dose of a betamimetic drug may be of value in some situations. Betamimetics administered with an inhaler or nebulizer do not abolish or reduce the uterine contractions effectively. Fetal scalp blood sampling (FBS) at the time of persistent prolonged deceleration, or soon after, may delay urgently needed action and is contraindicated.[2] Figure 13.2 shows the trace in a case without obvious risk factors. FBS, which can prolong the deceleration due to pressure on the fetal head, delayed delivery. CS was eventually performed. The baby had very poor Apgar scores and died on the third day of life after a period of neonatal convulsions.

Fetal acidosis observed soon after a prolonged deceleration (Fig. 13.3A) will recover when the trace returns to normal (Fig. 13.3B). However, if the FHR does not return to normal then delivery should be undertaken. During a prolonged deceleration the fetus reduces its cardiac output. Carbon dioxide and other metabolites cannot be cleared by the respiratory function of the placenta. The initial pH at the end of a prolonged deceleration is low with a high PCO_2 showing a respiratory acidosis. Once the FHR returns to normal, the carbon dioxide and metabolites are cleared and the pH as well as blood gases return to normal in 30–40 min. If the episode of prolonged deceleration continues then the fetus switches to anaerobic metabolism, resulting in metabolic acidosis, which is harmful to the fetus. Hence excessively prolonged deceleration results in a poor outcome.

Scar rupture or dehiscence may not show the classical symptoms and signs of scar pain, tenderness, vaginal bleeding or alteration in maternal pulse or blood pressure. Changes in FHR or uterine activity may be an earlier manifestation of loss of integrity of the scar, and prompt action should avoid fetal or maternal morbidity or mortality. In these cases, a prolonged deceleration may be an ominous sign and may indicate scar rupture. Figure 13.4A shows a prolonged deceleration in a case of labour with a previous CS. Delivery was

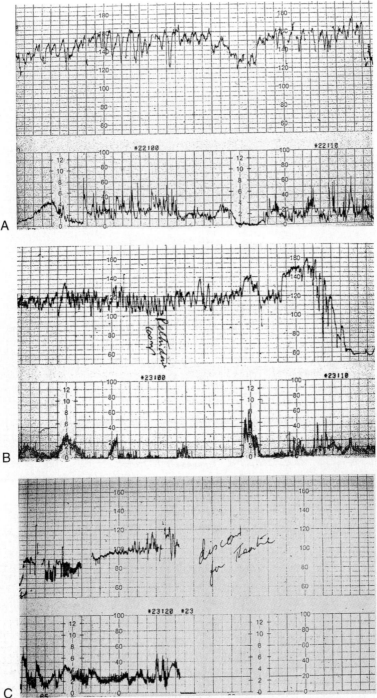

Fig. 13.1 ■ (A) Cardiotocograph: normal reactive pattern; (B) prolonged bradycardia; (C) improvement in heart rate.

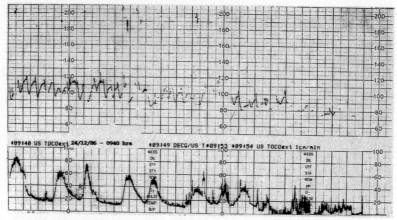

Fig. 13.2 ■ Fetal scalp blood sampling delays delivery: poor outcome.

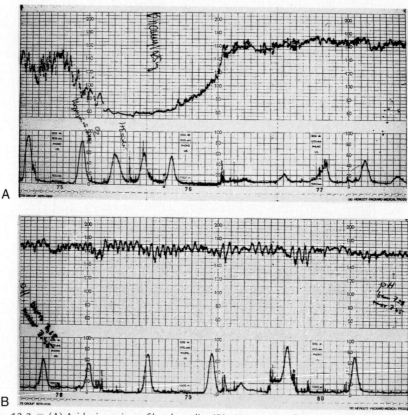

Fig. 13.3 ■ (A) Acidosis at time of bradycardia; (B) pH recovers after trace returns to normal.

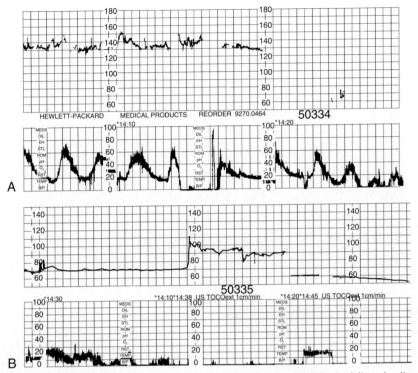

Fig. 13.4 ■ (A) Labour with previous caesarean section: prolonged bradycardia; (B) delay in delivery leading to poor outcome.

delayed (Fig. 13.4B), resulting in a baby with poor Apgar scores and neonatal asphyxial death on the second day. Whenever an operative delivery is planned, the fetal heart should be checked prior to delivery, as the baby may be already dead if there has been delay, but if scar rupture is suspected then CS needs to be done to repair the scar.

A prolonged deceleration following an eclamptic fit is shown in Figure 13.5. The convulsions were controlled and the baby was delivered in 30 min – a reasonable delay to stabilize the maternal condition. The fetal heart was not verified just before delivery and the baby was a fresh stillbirth.[3] In cases of placental abruption it may not be possible to listen to the fetal heart with a stethoscope or an electronic monitor. An ultrasound scan is therefore useful.

The procedure in the case of prolonged deceleration is shown in Table 13.1. Each hospital should have facilities to perform an immediate CS and deliver the baby within 15–20 min of taking the decision, especially in the case of high-risk labours (such as those of previous CS). This is referred to as delivery from a 'hot start'.

Delivery by CS from a 'cold start' may be permitted with a decision-to-delivery interval of 30 min. Audit and review of this in any unit is important.

THE DYING FETUS DUE TO GRADUALLY DEVELOPING HYPOXIA

Fetal death is always preceded by a terminal bradycardia. The trace with a normal FHR starts to show decelerations which may show increase in depth and duration of deceleration, reduction in intervals between decelerations with a rise in the baseline rate and a reduction in baseline variability before proceeding to a rapid stepwise drop in the baseline rate prior to the terminal bradycardia.

Figure 13.6A–J shows 10 sequential hourly traces in a mismanaged case of a high-risk mother suffering from sickle cell disease. This case occurred many years ago. The baby was known to be growth restricted with oligohydramnios. For reasons difficult to comprehend the medical staff failed to act and at delivery this baby was severely asphyxiated. The variable decelerations show increase

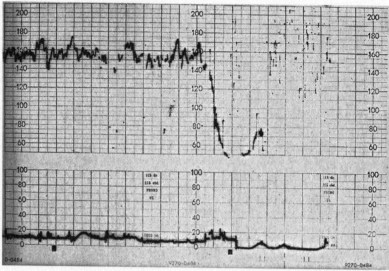

Fig. 13.5 ■ Prolonged bradycardia following eclamptic fit.

TABLE 13.1	
Procedure for Prolonged Bradycardia	
3 min	Draw attention and review clinical picture and prior fetal heart rate (FHR) trace
6 min	Expect recovery of FHR toward the baseline
9 min	If no recovery, prepare for operative delivery
12 min	Operative procedure should have started
15 min	Baby is delivered

in depth and duration with classical progression of the baseline rate to tachycardia, with no accelerations, and reduced variability for 1–2 h before the stepping down of the baseline FHR prior to terminal bradycardia. The baby was a fresh stillbirth. Knowing that the patient was a high-risk nulliparous woman, all who have read this book would have delivered the baby by the time of the third strip of tracing when there was normal baseline variability, Delivery of the baby at that time would have been in a reasonable condition. This high-risk woman had everything modern technology could offer, with the notable exception of basic common sense on the part of the staff.

'Chronic' or Pre-existing Hypoxia (Longstanding)

Some fetuses get compromised very slowly (chronic or longstanding) in the antenatal period and are at the verge of acute compromise with labour and show shallow

decelerations or are unable to generate decelerations due to the 'blunted response' by the hypoxic brain. This type of trace (Figs 13.7 and 13.8) is often misunderstood. There may be little in the way of a tachycardia but there is a complete absence of accelerations, a silent pattern of baseline variability and subtle, shallow late decelerations. This is an ominous picture and the baby must be delivered. These babies tend to have other clinical symptoms or signs such as absent fetal movements, intrauterine growth restriction (IUGR), intrauterine infection, bleeding, post-term pregnancy or scanty fluid with thick meconium.

An Ominous Tracing Demands Delivery

Birth asphyxia is often associated with pre-labour asphyxia. This highlights the value of the admission test whenever there is a suspicion of fetal compromise or in an unbooked case. Should all babies with ominous traces be delivered with the expectation of a living, undamaged child? We are obliged to deliver all such babies. It is difficult to know which babies will have a poor prognosis. Prognosis is poor if we procrastinate and deliver only when bradycardia sets in.

Pre-terminal FHR Patterns

Intervention in a fetus with a previously normal reactive trace within a reasonable period of the deterioration due to an acute event such as an abruption is likely to result in a good outcome, assuming a reasonable gestational age. Intervening when the main feature is

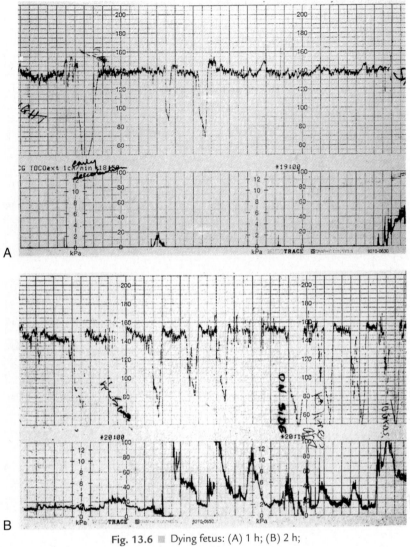

Fig. 13.6 ■ Dying fetus: (A) 1 h; (B) 2 h;

(continued)

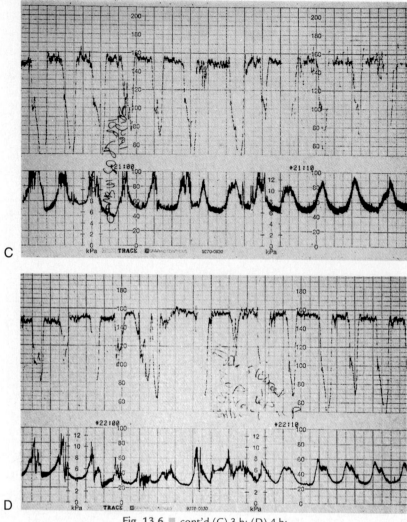

Fig. 13.6 ■ cont'd (C) 3 h; (D) 4 h;

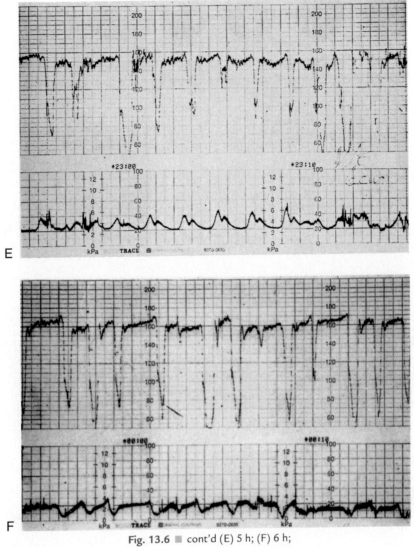

Fig. 13.6 ■ cont'd (E) 5 h; (F) 6 h;

(continued)

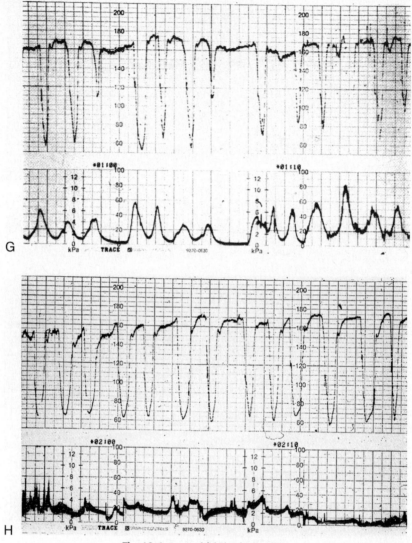

Fig. 13.6 ■ cont'd (G) 7 h; (H) 8 h;

(continued)

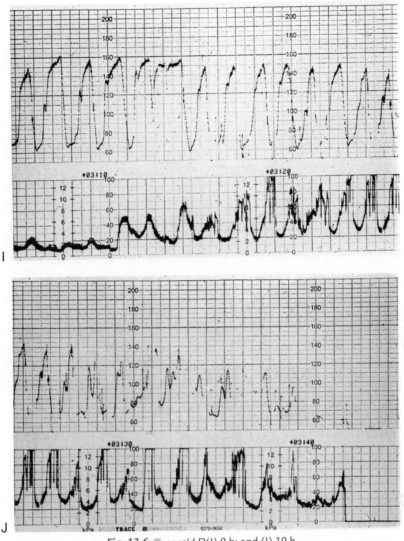

Fig. 13.6 ■ cont'd D(I) 9 h; and (J) 10 h.

tachycardia suggests some ability of the fetus to survive. Once the terminal bradycardia develops after the tachycardia the situation may be irretrievable (Fig. 13.9), especially when there are features of a random, uncontrolled undulatory pattern with no baseline variability (Fig. 13.10). This pattern suggests the possibility of central nervous system damage due to hypoxia. The challenge is to intervene in such pregnancies before this situation is reached; however, it should be kept in mind that central nervous system malformations can give rise to such patterns (see Ch. 7).

We are now in such a state of knowledge that the parents may be informed of the likelihood of a poor outcome despite intervention. For the moment, delivery remains mandatory.

RECORDING OF THE MATERNAL HEART RATE THAT CAN MIMIC THE FETAL HEART RATE

1. The MHR recording can mimic the FHR recording. This can arise in many situations and the

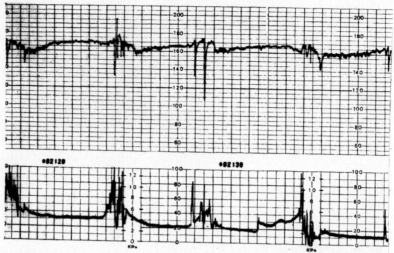

Fig. 13.7 ■ Ominous trace. Absent variability and shallow decelerations suggest pre-existing hypoxia.

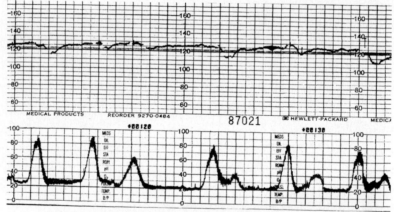

Fig. 13.8 ■ Ominous trace. Absent baseline variability and shallow decelerations despite the baseline rate being within the normal baseline heart rate. Accelerations and normal baseline variability are the hallmarks of fetal health. A normal baseline rate alone does not determine fetal health.

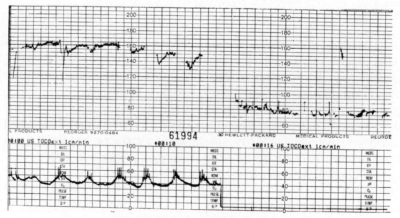

Fig. 13.9 ■ Terminal bradycardia.

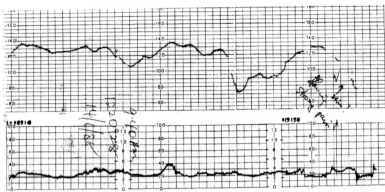

Fig. 13.10 ■ Terminal hypoxic central nervous system damage reflected by the inability to maintain a steady baseline rate and absent variability.

steps to avoid this are to follow the current recommendation of the Medical Devices Agency. At the onset of the electronic fetal monitoring auscultate the FHR and apply the transducer, rather than cross-checking with the maternal pulse. The reason for this is that the maternal pulse can be picked up by the ultrasound transducer and can be doubled (an increase of 100%), or it could be increased by 50%. It would be difficult to state whether the recording seen is that of the mother or the fetus.

2. It is also not uncommon for the machine to switch from fetal to MHR halfway through the recording. Any sudden shift in the baseline rate or a doubling of the baseline rate should indicate the possibility of recording the MHR and should warrant auscultation of the FHR.

3. Should there be a technically unsatisfactory recording with an ultrasound, it is important that a scalp electrode is applied to obtain continuous FHR recording unless there is a contraindication to the use of a fetal scalp electrode. This occurs more commonly in the late first and second stage of labour when the head moves down, or when the mother is restless, or there are too-frequent contractions with decelerations.

4. Be wary of a clear step change in the fetal heart pattern during the late first stage and the second stage of labour as the fetal head descends. This may not necessarily be a change in baseline rate, but rather a change in appearance (Fig. 13.11). The overall features of baseline variability and reactivity seen on a trace are consistent throughout labour allowing for the normal variation of fetal sleep/wake cycles. At this stage of labour, the baseline heart rates of mother and baby may be rather similar. The reappearance of accelerations, especially those that coincide with uterine contractions, is not reassuring after their preceding absence. It may be acceleration of the mother's heart (see below). Auscultation may help, but application of a fetal scalp electrode will clarify the picture.

The following gives an explanation of how these incidents occur. The characteristics of the MHR recording are different from those of the FHR recording in the second stage of labour. The FHR decelerates with head compression, while the MHR often increases with the uterine contractions. This should be identified and the FHR should be auscultated if there is any doubt. This knowledge should be disseminated widely to the maternity service practitioners (doctors and midwives). It would also be useful for those who are working in the community and midwifery birthing centres.

The Appearance of the Maternal Heart Rate in Labour

The traces shown in Figure 4.28 are simultaneous recordings of the FHR (upper trace) and MHR (middle trace). The MHR is recorded by a precordial electrocardiograph (ECG) lead on the anterior aspect of the mother's chest and is indicated automatically by the

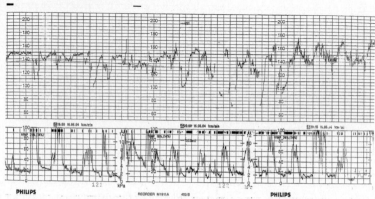

Fig. 13.11 ■ Observe the change in the fetal heart rate decelerative pattern with each contraction suddenly shifting to an accelerative pattern of maternal heart rate. The rise starts with the onset of the contractions and returns to its baseline rate with the offset of the contractions.

machine as 'MECG' in between the contraction (lower trace) and the FHR chart channels. The MHR recording shows features of accelerations and increased baseline variability.

Unless closely observed for the accelerations corresponding to the contractions it is similar to the FHR. The MHR pattern in labour has been studied.[4] Following such studies the unintentional recording of MHR in labour has been increasingly reported[4,5] and it has been shown that increase of the MHR with contractions is present in most cases. *This rise in the baseline heart rate may be a response to the increased blood flowing into the maternal heart during the uterine contractions.* A typical example is shown in Figure 13.11.

The CTG shown in Figure 2.6 was that of a dead fetus and the signals were recorded with the use of a scalp electrode, which shows the accelerations corresponding to the uterine contractions. In situations of fetal death, the ultrasound transducer may pick up one of the maternal vessel pulsations and present it on the recorder, which gives a false impression of the FHR. If the characteristics of the MHR are not recognized one may continue to record, thinking that it is the FHR, only to find that the baby is stillborn or in poor condition.

One has to think why the heart rate is accelerating with contractions in the late first and second stage of labour instead of having early or variable decelerations compatible with compression of the fetal head. Unfortunately, this is not common knowledge to clinicians, nurses or midwives and many interpret this as an FHR

trace with accelerations in the second stage of labour. Alternatively, they mistake the peak of the increase of the MHR to be the baseline FHR (if the MHR remains high for a longer duration) and the return of the MHR to its baseline rate as FHR decelerations.

Figure 13.12 illustrates how the FHR is recorded for continuous FHR monitoring. Mostly it is done using an ultrasound transducer or a scalp electrode. If the baby is dead, there is a possibility that the maternal ECG could be transmitted via the electrode and recorded on the chart, and for observers to believe that it may be the FHR. Similarly, the ultrasound transducer can pick up any pulsating maternal vessels, calculate the rate and record this on the chart, mimicking an FHR, especially when there is no FHR or a very low FHR.

Figure 13.13 illustrates how the ultrasound transducer can slip from its original position where it was picking up the fetal heart, and then pick up a maternal pulsation, giving a trace of the MHR that may appear like the FHR, unless someone recognizes it and readjusts the transducer to get the FHR. If it were not recognized, the MHR would have been recorded without knowledge of the FHR until the end of labour. Here the sudden shift is obvious, but in exceptional cases, it may be very subtle and difficult to pick up unless there is close scrutiny to observe the sudden changes in the baseline rate or the characteristics of the heart rate pattern.

It is known that the ultrasound transducer may pick up the maternal signal if the target signal moves away, such as after delivery of one twin or when there is sudden death of a fetus or acute fetal bradycardia.

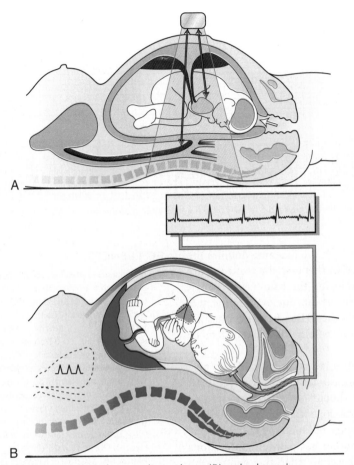

Fig. 13.12 ■ Recording fetal heart rate by (A) ultrasound transducer; (B) scalp electrode.

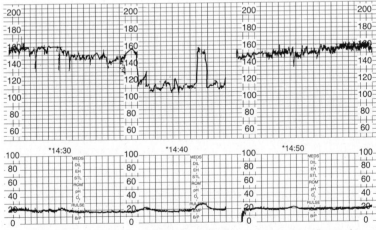

Fig. 13.13 ■ Recording by ultrasound – initial recording is that of the fetus. The ultrasound transducer slipped to the flank and picked up the maternal heart rate. This was identified and the transducer was replaced to record the fetal heart rate.

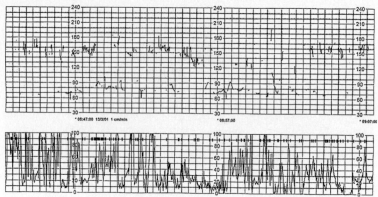

Fig. 13.14 ■ Trace showing fetal bradycardia of 70–75 bpm and doubling of the rate to 140–150 bpm thus giving two heart rates.

Figure 13.14 shows how the machine doubles the FHR with bradycardia. In this case the two rates are seen, the lower line showing the true baseline FHR and the upper one the heart rate due to doubling. It is important to auscultate the FHR when two rates are recorded so as to identify whether it could be fetal or maternal.

At times the machine can record the MHR (perhaps doubled) with occasional glimpses of the FHR at a lower rate.[6] One should observe the heart rate in relation to the contractions with the bearing-down efforts in the second stage of labour. If the heart rate increases when the mother has painful contractions and returns to the baseline after the contraction returns to the baseline, it is most likely to be the MHR because the FHR should decelerate with contractions due to head compression.

REFERENCES

[1] Ingemarsson I, Arulkumaran S, Ratnam SS. Single injection of terbutaline in term labor. 1. Effect on fetal pH in cases with prolonged bradycardia. Am J Obstet Gynecol 1985;153:859–65.

[2] National Institute for Health and Care Excellence (NICE). Intrapartum care for healthy women and their babies. NICE clinical guideline 190. 3 December 2014. Online. Available: https://www.nice.org.uk/guidance/cg190/resources/intrapartum-care-for-healthy-women-and-babies-35109866447557. [accessed 10.08.16].

[3] Arulkumaran S, Ratnam SS. Caesarean sections in the management of severe hypertensive disorders in pregnancy and eclampsia. Singapore J Obstet Gynecol 1988;19:61–6.

[4] International Federation of Obstetrics and Gynaecology (FIGO). Guidelines for the use of fetal monitoring. Int J Gynecol Obstet 1987;25:159–67.

[5] Murray ML. Maternal or fetal heart rate? Avoiding intrapartum misidentification. J Obstet Gynecol Neonatal Nurs 2004;33:93–104.

[6] Schiffrin BS. The CTG and the timing and mechanism of fetal neurological injuries. In: Arulkumaran S, Gardosi J, guest eds. Intrauterine surveillance of the fetus. Best Pract Res Clin Obstet Gynaecol 2004;18(3):467–78.

14 FETAL SCALP BLOOD SAMPLING

DONALD GIBB ■ SABARATNAM ARULKUMARAN

The availability of fetal scalp blood sampling (FBS) for the assessment of fetal scalp capillary blood pH and its application in practice vary enormously. The National Institute for Health and Care Excellence (NICE) guidelines have suggested the use of scalp pH in situations with a suspicious and/or pathological cardiotocograph (CTG) after due consideration to the clinical situation.[1] At times the clinical situation may demand early delivery rather than a scalp pH. In reality, junior doctors use scalp pH more when they have less experience of labour ward responsibilities. This is understandable as they have a greater anxiety with a less-developed degree of understanding. As they gain experience and use pH as a guide, they then understand better the associations of an abnormal and a normal pH and will need this reassurance less often. The process of scalp blood sampling is undignified and uncomfortable for the woman. This is not to say it should not be done if properly indicated. However, its value in modern practice has been challenged on the grounds that scalp capillary pH may not reflect the arterial pH, may be false if contaminated with amniotic fluid, may occasionally give rise to massive fetal haemorrhage, may inadvertently lead to leak of cerebrospinal fluid and may delay the urgently needed intervention.[2]

When the fetal heart rate (FHR) is reactive and normal, the chance of fetal acidosis is extremely low.[3-5] When the FHR is severely abnormal, such as with prolonged bradycardia indicating acute hypoxia (described in Ch. 13) or repeated prolonged decelerations suggestive of sub-acute hypoxia (described in this chapter), the pH declines so rapidly that an immediate delivery is warranted and performing a pH is a waste of valuable time. All suspicious and abnormal FHR changes are not associated with acidosis.[4-7] Such observations form the basis of the perceived need to measure fetal scalp pH for further investigation. But this need has to be judged against the clinical picture of parity, current cervical dilatation, rate of progress, pyrexia, meconium and a growth-restricted baby where the physiological reserve is reduced. Consideration of these clinical issues provides a common-sense approach whether to deliver or to perform a pH with the understanding that more time can be given for the labour to progress and deliver vaginally if the pH is normal.

Changes in the CTG cause anxiety to the person not familiar with CTG interpretation. An inexperienced person in a centre with FBS facilities might perform FBS more frequently. When properly interpreted, assessment of FHR changes in most cases proves of equal value to pH in predicting fetal outcome.[8] FBS is a useful adjunct because, even with the worst pattern of tachycardia, reduced baseline variability and decelerations, only 50-60% of the fetuses are acidotic.[4] A wall chart correlating different FHR patterns to the percentage who are likely to be acidotic is available in most labour wards. It is clear from that chart and other studies that when the FHR pattern exhibited accelerations the chance of fetal acidosis was zero, emphasizing accelerations as the hallmark of fetal health.[4] One problem of these charts is that all fetuses do not conveniently provide a fetal heart tracing that easily falls into one particular category. There is the added perspective of the need for a time continuum, which is so important in trace analysis. The physiological reserve of some fetuses will show more decline in pH with one CTG trace rather than others (e.g., an appropriately grown fetus compared to one with intrauterine growth restriction [IUGR]).

Baseline variability, usually associated with accelerations, is another good indicator of fetal health. When normal baseline variability is observed in the last 20 minutes (min) prior to delivery, the babies are in good condition at birth regardless of other features of the trace.[9] Fetal acidosis is more common when there is a loss of baseline variability with tachycardia and late decelerations.[4,10] The preservation of normal baseline variability indicates that the autonomic nervous system is responsive and the fetus is trying to compensate despite other abnormal features in the trace. The reason that, with a given FHR pattern, there are varying numbers of fetuses showing acidosis depends on the duration for which the suspicious or abnormal FHR pattern was present before the time of FBS and the 'physiological reserve' of the fetus.[11] The approximate duration after which acidosis develops in an appropriately grown term fetus with a given FHR pattern has been discussed previously. It is also known that, in fetuses with less 'placental reserve' such as those with IUGR, thick, scanty meconium-stained fluid,[12] in the presence of bleeding and in post-term infants, the rate of decline of pH is steep compared with term infants appropriately grown with abundant, clear amniotic fluid. The consideration of the need for delivery is based on these clinical factors when the CTG is suspicious. An alternative would be assessing fetal scalp pH if labour is allowed to continue. When the trace is normal (presence of reactivity and cycling), there is no need for scalp pH or delivery; and when the trace is grossly abnormal with prolonged deceleration or sub-acute hypoxic pattern described in this chapter, or a trace with absent variability and late or atypical variable decelerations, there is a need for delivery; and performing a scalp pH will delay the delivery and worsen the condition of the fetus.

RESPIRATORY AND METABOLIC ACIDOSIS

Assessment of pH alone does not suffice to identify the fetus at risk, and more comprehensive blood gas analysis may be necessary for clinical management.

The placenta is the respiratory organ of the fetus. Reduction of perfusion of the placenta from the fetal circulation is manifest as variable decelerations due to cord compression, and reduction of perfusion from the maternal circulation is manifest as late decelerations. During the early stage of such threats the transfer of carbon dioxide from the fetal to maternal side is reduced, leading to its accumulation. This results in respiratory acidosis manifested by a low pH and a high PCO_2. Respiratory acidosis is transitory, and can be managed with corrective conservative measures (left lateral position, cessation of oxytocin infusion, hydration) and one could await for improvement of the FHR pattern.

With a further reduction of perfusion from the maternal or fetal side the oxygen transfer becomes affected, leading to anaerobic metabolism and metabolic acidosis in the fetus. This is manifested by a low pH, low PO_2 and high base excess. Such metabolic acidosis is damaging to the tissues. Transitory low pH values of respiratory type are not uncommon in low-risk labours. Acidotic pH values in cord arterial blood in babies born with good Apgar scores are due to this phenomenon: 73% of babies with cord pH below 7.00 had a 1 min Apgar score of more than 7, and 86% had a 5 min Apgar score greater than 7.[13] These findings are probably due to respiratory acidosis, which does not correlate well with the fetal or neonatal condition. In this situation, a comprehensive blood gas analysis, including PCO_2, base excess and preferably lactic acid, is desirable and more predictive. Caution should be exercised in using equipment that measures only pH. It is possible to determine the degree of metabolic acidosis by measuring the lactic acid level by the bedside with 5 μl of blood using the lactate card.[14] Intrauterine infection with a high metabolic rate presents a greater oxygen demand to the fetus, and metabolic acidosis might develop with minimal interruption of placental perfusion. This is not implemented commonly.

WHEN TO DO FETAL BLOOD SAMPLING

Gradually Developing Hypoxia (See Ch.13)

The fetus becomes hypoxic and acidotic in labour in association with compromise of perfusion to the fetal or maternal side of the placental circulation. With the exception of situations of acute hypoxia due to cord prolapse, scar dehiscence, abruption and prolonged deceleration, it is unusual for a fetus who has shown accelerations and good baseline variability to become hypoxic without developing decelerations in labour. The decelerations indicate the presence of stress to the fetus, whether from the challenge of poor perfusion or from mechanical pressure. Provided that the baseline FHR has not started to rise and there is no reduction in the baseline variability to less than 5 beats, there is little to be gained by performing FBS, as the pH is likely to be normal unless the decelerations are prolonged and last for a duration two to three times greater than the duration spent at the baseline FHR between the decelerations. If the baseline FHR has risen by 20–30 beats and is not showing any further rise, with a reduction in variability to less than 5 beats, then hypoxia is probable. Despite the fetus having increased its cardiac output to a possible maximum by increasing the FHR, the functioning of the autonomic nervous system controlling the baseline variability is compromised by hypoxia. The time course of this process may be referred to as the *stress-to-distress period*. This period varies from fetus to fetus depending on the physiological reserve. This reserve is low in high-risk situations of prolonged pregnancy, IUGR and intrauterine infection and in those with bleeding or thick meconium and scanty amniotic fluid.

When the FHR shows hypoxic features suggestive of distress (gradual increase of baseline rate, reduced baseline variability and increasing depth and duration of deceleration and often reduction of inter-deceleration intervals) it is important to perform FBS for pH and blood gases as the fetus may be, or become, acidotic. Initially this will be respiratory, followed by a metabolic acidosis. Once the FHR shows a distress pattern (markedly reduced baseline variability with late or atypical variable decelerations), the time taken for metabolic acidosis to develop is unpredictable. This pattern is referred to as a *preterminal pattern* by some authors. After a certain duration of the distress pattern (the *distress period*) the FHR starts to decline in a rapid stepwise pattern, culminating in terminal bradycardia and death (the *distress-to-death period*). The stress-to-distress interval (20.00–00.00 hours (h), i.e., 4 h), the distress period (00.00–03.00 h, i.e., 3 h) and the

distress-to-death period (03.00–03.40 h, i.e., 40 min) are illustrated in Figure 13.6A–J. Another example where the stress-to-distress period, the distress period and the distress-to-death period are much shorter is shown in Figure 8.4A–F. Clinical interpretation of the FHR pattern will identify the onset of stress, distress and the stress-to-distress period. It will also identify the fetus in the distress period. An accurate prediction of the distress period cannot be made based on the FHR pattern, as illustrated by these two examples. During the final decline phase (distress-to-death period), when the FHR drops irretrievably within a short period, it is often too late to intervene.

The value of FBS may be at the onset of the distress period and again repeated 30–40 min later or earlier, depending on the first pH and base excess, baseline variability and the type of decelerations. Adherence to the recommendation of immediate delivery when the pH is less than 7.20 (acidosis), and a repeat sample after 30 min or less when the pH was 7.20–7.25 (preacidosis) is good practice. Previous recommendations were that when the pH was greater than 7.25 the repeat sampling was not required unless the FHR deteriorated. This approach may generate a false sense of security when the trace does not deteriorate, although the pH is declining. Repeat measurement in appropriate time, based on the first pH and increasing abnormality of the trace (further rise in baseline rate, deepening and widening of the decelerations and reduction of the duration of the FHR at the baseline rate and reduction in baseline variability) even when the first pH is in the normal range, helps to identify the rate of decline.[15] A decision for delivery can be made considering the rate of decline of the pH, the clinical risk factors (IUGR, thick meconium), parity, current cervical dilatation and rate of progress of labour.

Sub-Acute Hypoxia

The pH may deteriorate rapidly in a fetus who had previously had a reactive trace without an increase in the baseline FHR, if the decelerations are pronounced with large dip areas (drop of more than 60 beats per min [bpm] for over 90 seconds [s]) with the FHR recovering to the baseline for only short periods of time (less than 60 s). Examples of such traces are shown in Figure 14.1A–F. In these situations a drop in pH can be by as much as 0.01 every 3–4 min. This decline in pH will be even steeper if the preceding trace was suspicious or abnormal, or the clinical picture was one of high risk (IUGR, thick meconium with scanty fluid or intrauterine infection). Further insults at this time, such as oxytocin infusion or a difficult instrumental delivery, may make the situation worse. With such traces, attempts at FBS will delay much-needed urgent delivery.

Chronic ('Long-Standing') Hypoxia

A non-reactive FHR pattern showing a baseline variability less than 5 beats with shallow decelerations (less than 15 beats for 15 s), even with a normal baseline rate, indicates severe compromise and delivery should be expedited without delay to avoid fetal death (see Fig. 8.6A–D). A non-reactive trace with a baseline variability of less than 5 beats but without decelerations lasting more than 90 min indicates the possibility of already existing hypoxic compromise or damage due to other reasons (e.g., cerebral haemorrhage). This needs further evaluation if the pH is normal. In these circumstances, fetal death may occur suddenly without further warning of a rise in baseline FHR or

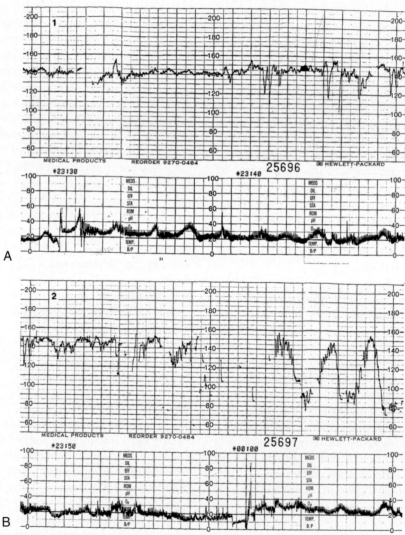

Fig. 14.1 ■ (A–F) Sub-acute hypoxia – prolonged decelerations (>90 s, depth >60 bpm) with short intervals of recovery (<60 s) to baseline rate.

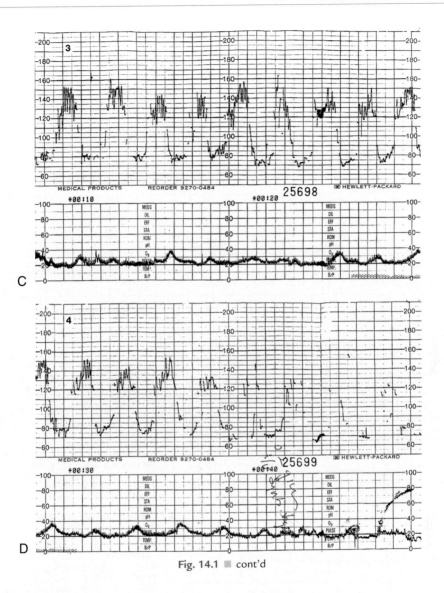

C

D

Fig. 14.1 ▪ cont'd

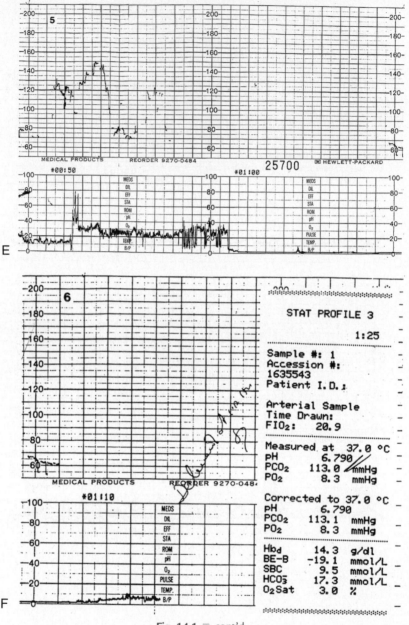

STAT PROFILE 3

1:25

Sample #: 1
Accession #:
1635543
Patient I.D.:

Arterial Sample
Time Drawn:
FIO₂: 20.9

Measured at 37.0 °C
pH   6.790
PCO₂   113.0   mmHg
PO₂   8.3   mmHg

Corrected to 37.0 °C
pH   6.790
PCO₂   113.1   mmHg
PO₂   8.3   mmHg

Hb_d   14.3   g/dl
BE-B   -19.1   mmol/L
SBC   9.5   mmol/L
HCO₃⁻   17.3   mmol/L
O₂Sat   3.0   %

Fig. 14.1 ▪ cont'd

decelerations (see Fig. 8.5A–J). Hence, a non-reactive trace for greater than 90 min is abnormal and is an indication for further evaluation to rule out hypoxia.

Acute Hypoxia

Abruption, cord prolapse, scar dehiscence and uterine hyper-stimulation may give rise to acute hypoxia. This may manifest as prolonged deceleration; at other times, prolonged deceleration occurs without obvious reason and in all circumstances is associated with rapidly progressive acidosis. With a bradycardia of less than 80 bpm the pH is likely to decline at the rate of approximately 0.01 per min.[16] The decline may be steeper in the presence of an abnormal trace prior to the bradycardia.

With FHR patterns suggestive of acute or sub-acute hypoxia, performing a FBS might delay intervention, resulting in poor outcome. In FHR patterns with poor variability lasting for more than 90 min, but with no decelerations, investigations should be performed to identify the cause. The principle can be established that the FHR pattern identifies the onset of stress (decelerations) and of distress (maximal elevation of baseline FHR with baseline variability less than 5 beats). Although the onset of stress and distress can be identified, the duration of the distress period before the fetus becomes hypoxic and acidotic cannot be predicted. A decision is required to deliver or to perform FBS, bearing in mind the clinical picture, if the prospect of early delivery is poor.

WHEN NOT TO DO FETAL BLOOD SAMPLING

Frequently the FHR changes observed might be due to factors other than hypoxia. Dehydration, ketosis, maternal pyrexia and anxiety can give rise to fetal tachycardia but do not usually present with decelerations. Occipitoposterior position is known to be associated with more variable decelerations without hypoxic features, as evidenced by normal baseline rate and variability.[17] Oxytocin can cause hyper-stimulation resulting in FHR changes of various forms, which have been discussed in Chapter 10. Prolonged bradycardia can be due to postural hypotension following epidural analgesia. FHR changes should be correlated with the clinical picture before action is taken.

In many instances remedial actions such as hydration, repositioning of the mother or stopping the oxytocin infusion will relieve the FHR changes and no further action is necessary. When the FHR changes persist despite such actions, a FBS or one of the stimulation tests is warranted. At times FBS may not be necessary because the trace is reassuring with accelerations and normal baseline variability despite some decelerations (see Fig. 14.4), or it may show a low result transiently and later a good result; the pH may be low transiently owing to respiratory acidosis. Above all, when the trace is ominous or the clinical picture is poor it is better to deliver the baby rather than wasting time with an FBS. At times a false reassurance leads to an unsatisfactory outcome.

Fetal blood sampling is not appropriate under the following circumstances:

1. When the clinical picture demands early delivery (Fig. 14.2): 42 weeks gestation, cervix 3 cm dilated, thick meconium with scanty fluid.
2. When an ominous trace prompts immediate delivery (Fig. 14.3).
3. When the FHR trace is reassuring (Fig. 14.4).
4. When the changes are due to oxytocic overstimulation (see Fig. 10.5).
5. When there is associated persistent failure to progress in labour (Fig. 14.5).
6. During, or soon after, an episode of prolonged bradycardia (see Fig. 10.4).
7. If spontaneous vaginal delivery is imminent or easy instrumental vaginal delivery is possible (see Fig. 12.14).

Following these principles will help to avoid unnecessary FBS, operative deliveries and fetal morbidity from undue delay in delivery.

ALTERNATIVES TO FETAL BLOOD SAMPLING FOR pH

Measurement of lactate in scalp blood is becoming more popular especially in Scandinavian countries because of the small blood samples required for analysis (5 μl instead of 35 μl for pH and base excess). This leads to a failure rate for sampling of 2%–4% compared with 15%–18% with scalp sampling for pH. It also has

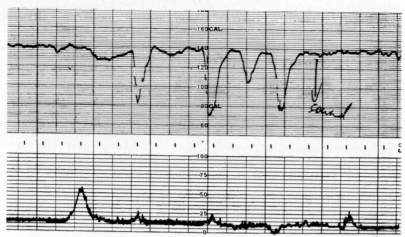

Fig. 14.2 ■ Clinical picture demands early delivery.

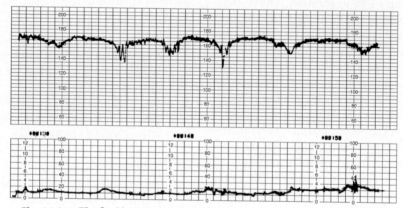

Fig. 14.3 ■ The fetal heart rate trace is ominous prompting immediate delivery.

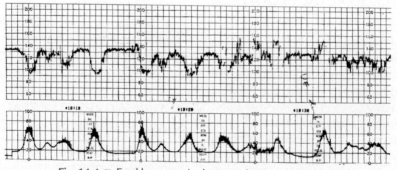

Fig. 14.4 ■ Fetal heart rate in the second stage – reassuring.

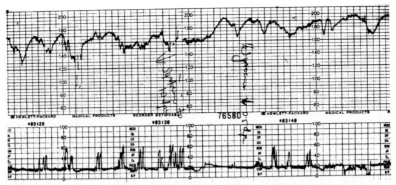

Fig. 14.5 ■ Changes in fetal heart rate – failure to progress in labour.

an impact on the time needed for sampling. Caput formation does not alter the correlation between scalp and circulatory values. Lactate levels increase in the mother and the fetus in the second stage of labour throughout the period of bearing-down efforts – the lactate levels increase by 1 mmol/l every 30 min. Studies have shown a good correlation between the scalp and cord lactate when the sampling intervals have been close. The normal values for lactate vary based on the machine used (Lactate Pro or Accuport). Using the Lactate Pro machine, a value of less than 4.2 mmol/l is considered normal and a repeat performance is needed only if the CTG abnormalities persist or get worse; a value of 4.2–4.8 is considered intermediate needing a repeat estimation within 30 min; and greater than 4.8 is considered abnormal and an indication for immediate delivery.

In practice, FBS for pH or lactate may not be performed because the facilities or the expertise is not available, or because it is technically difficult. Alternative indirect methods are useful in this situation. A retrospective observation and correlation of the scalp blood pH to the presence or absence of accelerations at the time of FBS (Fig. 14.6) led to the *scalp stimulation test*.[18] When the scalp was stimulated by pinching with a tissue forceps, if an acceleration was present it was unlikely that the scalp blood pH was below 7.20.[19,20] In contrast, if there were no accelerations to such a stimulus then only about 50% had acidotic pH values (<7.20), whereas a significant proportion had preacidotic values (7.20–7.25) and others had normal values (Table 14.1).

Therefore, this test was useful in identifying those who are not at risk, although it was not good in predicting those who are likely to be acidotic. In centres where facilities do not exist for scalp FBS, such a test would be a useful adjunct in reducing the number of unnecessary caesarean sections for 'fetal distress', and in centres where facilities are available for FBS it will reduce the number of samples taken. Where there is a failure to obtain a sample during the FBS procedure, observation of an acceleration is very reassuring and the procedure can be discontinued.

In the study described above, the case that recorded a positive response with an acidotic pH (see Table 14.1) showed respiratory acidosis, which is due to accumulation of CO_2, is not harmful to the fetus and is known to reverse itself once the FHR returns to normal. Careful observation of the characteristics of the FHR resulted in a fetus born with good Apgar scores. The latest NICE guideline also endorses the view that if FBS fails but digital stimulation provokes an acceleration then the situation needs to be reviewed.[1]

The Royal College of Obstetricians and Gynaecologists Study Group[21] and NICE have recommended that FBS facilities should be available in any hospital where electronic fetal monitoring is performed. However, clinicians who understand the clinical situation and the FHR pattern may make a decision without resorting to FBS and without an increase in caesarean section rate for fetal distress.[22] In many situations it may be wiser to proceed to delivery without wasting precious time. It has been shown that if the decision-to-delivery interval in situations of fetal distress is 35 min as opposed to 15 min then the admission rate to the neonatal intensive care unit is doubled.[23] FBS is not always possible because facilities may not be available, or it may be difficult to perform owing to an undilated cervix or high

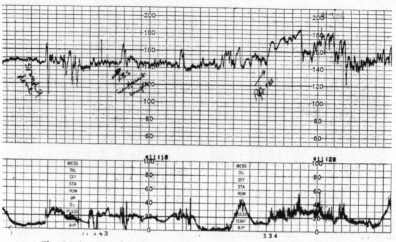

Fig. 14.6 ■ Acceleration at fetal scalp blood sampling – normal pH.

TABLE 14.1

Results of Scalp Stimulation Tests in Relation to Scalp Blood pH Values[20]

Response to Scalp Stimulation	Fetal Scalp Blood pH Values			
	<7.20 (n = 82)	7.20–7.25 (n = 156)	>7.25 (n = 462)	Total (n = 700)
Positive response	1 (0.4%)	33 (12.7%)	226 (86.9%)	260
Negative response	40 (44.4%)	45 (50.0%)	5 (5.6%)	90
Total	41 (11.7%)	78 (22.3%)	231 (66%)	350

head.[24,25] In these situations, decisions based on the CTG and the clinical situation remain critical.

POINTS TO PONDER

Although pH is a useful adjunct, the following points should be considered in clinical decision-making:[26]

- Accelerations and normal baseline variability are hallmarks of fetal health.
- Accelerations without baseline variability should be considered suspicious.
- Periods of decreased baseline variability without decelerations may represent quiet fetal sleep.
- Hypoxic fetuses may have a normal baseline FHR of 110–160 bpm with no accelerations and baseline variability less than 5 bpm for greater than 40 min (in the absence of adverse clinical parameters, observation for greater than 90 min may be needed to recognize the abnormality).

- In the presence of baseline variability of less than 5 bpm, even shallow decelerations of less than 15 bpm are ominous in a non-reactive trace.
- Abruption, cord prolapse and scar rupture can cause acute hypoxia and should be suspected clinically (may give rise to prolonged decelerations/bradycardia).
- Fetal hypoxia and acidosis may develop faster with an abnormal trace when there is scanty, thick meconium, bleeding, IUGR, intrauterine infection with pyrexia and/or pre- or post-term labour.
- In pre-term fetuses (especially <34 weeks), hypoxia and acidosis can increase the likelihood of respiratory distress syndrome and may contribute to intraventricular haemorrhage, warranting early intervention in the presence of an abnormal trace.
- Hypoxia can be made worse by injudicious use of oxytocin, epidural analgesia and difficult operative deliveries.

- During labour, if decelerations are absent, asphyxia is unlikely although it cannot be completely excluded.
- Abnormal patterns may represent the effects of drugs, fetal anomaly, fetal injury or infection – not only hypoxia.

REFERENCES

[1] National Institute for Health and Care Excellence (NICE). Intrapartum care for healthy women and their babies. NICE clinical guideline 190; 3. 2014. Online. Available: https://www.nice.org.uk/guidance/cg190/resources/intrapartum-care-for-healthy-women-and-babies-35109866447557. [accessed 10.08.16].

[2] Chandraharan E. Fetal scalp blood sampling during labour: is it a useful diagnostic test or a historical test that no longer has a place in modern clinical obstetrics? BJOG 2014;121:1056–62.

[3] Beard RW, Morris ED, Clayton SG. pH of fetal capillary blood as an indicator of the condition of the fetus. J Obstet Gynaecol Br Commonw 1967;74:812–7.

[4] Beard RW, Filshie GM, Knight CA, et al. The significance of the changes in the continuous fetal heart rate in the first stage of labour. J Obstet Gynaecol Br Commonw 1971;78:865–81.

[5] Ingemarsson E. Routine electronic fetal monitoring during labor. Acta Obstet Gynecol Scand 1981;99:1–29.

[6] Zalor RW, Quilligan EJ. The influence of scalp sampling on the caesarean section rate for fetal distress. Am J Obstet Gynecol 1979;135:239–46.

[7] Katz M, Mazor M, Insler V. Fetal heart rate patterns and scalp pH as predictors of fetal distress. Isr J Med Sci 1981;17:260–5.

[8] Parer JT. In defense of FHR monitoring's specificity. Cont Obstet Gynaecol 1982;19:228–34.

[9] Paul RH, Suidan AK, Yeh SY, et al. Clinical fetal monitoring. VII. The evaluation and significance of intrapartum baseline variability. Am J Obstet Gynecol 1975;123:206–10.

[10] Schifrin BS, Dame L. Fetal heart rate patterns: prediction of Apgar score. JAMA 1972;219:1322–5.

[11] Fleischer A, Schulman H, Jagani N, et al. The development of fetal acidosis in the presence of an abnormal fetal heart rate tracing. I. The average for gestation age fetus. Am J Obstet Gynecol 1982;144:55–60.

[12] Starks GC. Correlation of meconium stained amniotic fluid, early intrapartum fetal pH and Apgar scores as predictors of perinatal outcome. Obstet Gynecol 1980;55:604–9.

[13] Sykes GS, Molloy PM, Johnson P, et al. Do Apgar scores indicate asphyxia? Lancet 1982;1(8270):494–6.

[14] Nordstrom L, Arulkumaran S, Chua S, et al. Continuous maternal glucose infusion during labor: effects on maternal and fetal glucose and lactate levels. Am J Perinatol 1995;12:357–62.

[15] Huch A, Huch R, Rooth G. Guidelines for blood sampling and measurements of pH and blood gas values in obstetrics. Eur J Obstet Gynecol Reprod Biol 1994;54:165–75.

[16] Arulkumaran S, Yang M, Chia YT, et al. Reliability of intrauterine pressure measurements. Obstet Gynecol 1991;78:800–2.

[17] Ingemarsson I, Ingemarsson E, Solum T, et al. Influence of occiput posterior position on the fetal heart rate pattern. Obstet Gynecol 1980;55:301–6.

[18] Clarke SL, Gimovsky ML, Miller FC. Fetal heart rate response to scalp blood sampling. Am J Obstet Gynecol 1983;144:706–8.

[19] Clarke SL, Gimovsky ML, Miller FC. The scalp stimulation test: a clinical alternative to fetal scalp blood sampling. Am J Obstet Gynecol 1984;148:274–7.

[20] Arulkumaran S, Ingemarsson I, Ratnam SS. Fetal heart rate response to scalp stimulation as a test for fetal wellbeing in labour. Asia-Oceania J Obstet Gynecol 1987;13:131–5.

[21] Recommendations arising from the 26th royal College of Obstetricians and Gynaecologists (RCOG) study group. In: Spencer JAD, editor. Intrapartum fetal surveillance. London: RCOG Press; 1993. p. 387–93.

[22] Clarke SL, Paul RH. Intrapartum fetal surveillance: the role of fetal scalp blood sampling. Am J Obstet Gynecol 1985;153:717–20.

[23] Dunphy BC, Robinson JN, Sheil OM, et al. Caesarean section for fetal distress, the interval from decision to delivery, and the relative risk of poor neonatal condition. Br J Obstet Gynaecol 1991;11:241–4.

[24] Gillmer MDG, Combe D. Intrapartum fetal monitoring practice in the United Kingdom. Br J Obstet Gynaecol 1979;86:753–8.

[25] Wheble AM, Gillmer MDG, Spencer JAD, et al. Changes in fetal monitoring practice in the UK: 1977–1984. Br J Obstet Gynaecol 1989;96:1140–7.

[26] Arulkumaran S, Montan S, Ingemarsson I, et al. Traces of you – fetal trace interpretation. Best, Netherlands: Philips Medical Systems; 2002. Ref. 4522 981 88671/862.

15

FETAL ELECTROCARDIOGRAPH WAVEFORM ANALYSIS

AUSTIN UGWUMADU

The incidence of neonatal, childhood and longer-term morbidity and mortality arising during labour has remained relatively static in the UK and other developed countries. This is in spite of decades of the use of the cardiotocograph (CTG) with adjunctive fetal scalp blood sample (FBS) for pH or lactate measurements for intrapartum fetal surveillance. However, these tools and their operational guidelines are focused on detecting intrapartum oxygen deprivation and hypoxic ischaemic insults but make no recommendations on other noxious but non-hypoxia related factors, which are also associated with fetal injury such as maternal fever, chorioamnionitis, fetal host inflammatory response and its synergistic interaction with hypoxia, abnormal behavioural states, excessive head moulding and fetal strokes, to name a few. Therefore a fetal surveillance system that captures these varied insult paradigms and/or is focused on the final common pathway to injury is warranted. Studies in Scandinavian countries using specific lesions on magnetic resonance imaging (MRI) suggest that intrapartum asphyxia, either de novo or exacerbating pre-existing insult, is the likely cause of cerebral palsy in up to 28% of children with cerebral palsy who were born at term.[1,2]

In 2015 the Royal College of Obstetricians and Gynaecologists launched a quality improvement programme 'Each Baby Counts' to examine the factors which underlie term stillbirths especially in the intrapartum period and learn how to avoid them.[3] In 2016 National Health Service England launched a care bundle approach to reduce stillbirths, and one of the components of the bundle is training and assessment of intrapartum fetal surveillance.[4] The current state of training and certification in intrapartum fetal heart rate (FHR) monitoring is in a flux,[5] and we need to improve our methods of surveillance and actions based on them if we are to avoid intrapartum-related morbidity and mortality. Fetal electrocardiograph (ECG) waveform analysis (STAN) was introduced to reduce perinatal morbidity and mortality in the 1990s. The fetal myocardium is a high-priority organ and receives increased blood flow and oxygen delivery in times of hypoxic or other stressors.

ASSESSMENT OF THE BRAIN AND THE HEART BY COMBINED CTG AND ECG WAVEFORM ANALYSIS

FHR accelerations occur with fetal movements and suggest integrity of the 'somatic' nervous system. Normal baseline FHR variability suggests integrity of the 'autonomic' nervous system. Decelerations are reflex cardiovascular responses to brief interruption of oxygen delivery to the fetus and relate to mechanisms that may cause hypoxia.[6] Therefore the CTG assesses the integrity of the fetal nervous system, whilst the ST changes of T-wave or ST segment elevation and/or distortion reflect the strain to the heart. Hence a combination of both parameters gives information on hypoxic stress to the heart and the brain. When all four features of the CTG trace are normal, the chance of fetal acidosis is small. When all the features are abnormal, just over 50% are noted to be acidotic.[7] The clinician may respond differently to hypoxic insults depending on the physiological reserve of the fetus. Fleischer et al. showed that, for 50% of appropriately grown term fetuses in spontaneous labour with clear amniotic fluid and normal CTG to become acidotic, it takes 115 minutes (min) with repetitive late decelerations, 145 min with repetitive variable decelerations and 185 min with a 'flat trace' (i.e., with reduced baseline variability).[8] This suggests that some fetuses may become acidotic within a shorter period of time, more so if there is reduced physiological reserve due to infection, bleeding, post-term or growth restriction and in those with scanty thick meconium-stained fluid. Therefore it is important to determine the fetal condition and need for operative delivery when there are abnormal FHR changes by FBS or other appropriate alternative technology. However, the facilities and expertise to perform FBS are not available in many centres.[9,10] Fetuses with infection and FHR tachycardia have an increased risk of encephalopathy and cerebral palsy without acidaemia or bradycardia,[11] suggesting direct neurologic injury by inflammation or other non-hypoxia pathway. There are no differences in acid base status between infected and noninfected fetuses, but infected fetuses have significantly lower Apgar scores.[12] A paradoxic discrepancy exists between the need for FBS and when one is done in practice.[13] The intermittent nature of FBS readings makes it difficult to identify the optimal time to intervene without compromising the fetus, and without increasing operative interventions. These issues have prompted more units to turn to the use ECG–ST waveform analysis for fetal surveillance in labour because Cochrane reviews of available studies have shown a significant reduction of FBS and operative vaginal deliveries with the use of STAN.

FETAL ECG–ST WAVEFORM ANALYSIS

Fetal ECG waveform analysis relies on computerised analysis of changes in the ST segment of the fetal ECG as they relate to metabolic events in the fetal myocardium during hypoxia. Recent advances in biomedical engineering, computer processing power and animal experimental data have resulted in progress in the computerised analysis of the ST waveform. The ST analyser STAN (Neoventa, Gotenborg, Sweden) is a CTG machine, which provides a CTG trace. When the

FHR signals are obtained using an internal scalp electrode on the fetal scalp and a skin reference electrode on the maternal thigh, it provides fetal ECG ST waveform analysis. Animal experimental data have demonstrated a catecholamine surge with hypoxic stress. This results in mobilisation of stored myocardial glycogen. This important defence mechanism of adrenoceptor stimulation[14] brings about a shift in glucose and K^+ ions leading to increased T-wave amplitude (T/QRS ratio) (Fig. 15.1A and B). The detection of ST changes is computerized and the STAN equipment highlights any significant changes in the ST segment. The ST events detected may be (i) a *baseline rise* of the T/QRS ratio, (ii) an *episodic rise* of the T/QRS ratio or (iii) a *biphasic ST* segment. Each fetus has a stable T/QRS ratio in early labour that could be identified from the initial recording. The rise in the T/QRS ratio is calculated with reference to the lowest T/QRS ratio calculated over the initial 20 averaged T/QRS complexes, which takes no longer than 5–10 min to establish and presented in the event log. Therefore the equipment needs to be used for 5–10 min to calculate the baseline T/QRS ratio prior to major changes in heart rate. A *preterminal trace* that shows total lack of baseline variability and reactivity, with or without decelerations, or a persistently prolonged deceleration warrants immediate delivery.

A steadily increasing T/QRS rise for greater than 10 min is termed a *baseline rise,* and if the ratio increases significantly and comes down in less than 10 min, it is termed an *episodic rise.* The biphasic event refers to alteration of the morphology of the ST segment where there is an initial rise and then a fall (Fig. 15.2). If the ST change is above the isoelectric line (the horizontal line constructed based on the resting level of the P wave), it is termed biphasic 1; if it cuts the isoelectric line, it is called biphasic 2; and if it is below the isoelectric line, it is called biphasic 3. Biphasic 2 and 3 are considered significant and are related to the flow of electrical current between the endocardium and the epicardium. These changes may be present in the following situations: when the myocardium is thin (e.g., preterm fetuses), and when there is myocardial disease, infection and hypoxia.[15] The FHR pattern, the ECG complex with T/QRS analysis and uterine contractions are recorded onscreen on the same trace as shown in Figure 15.3.

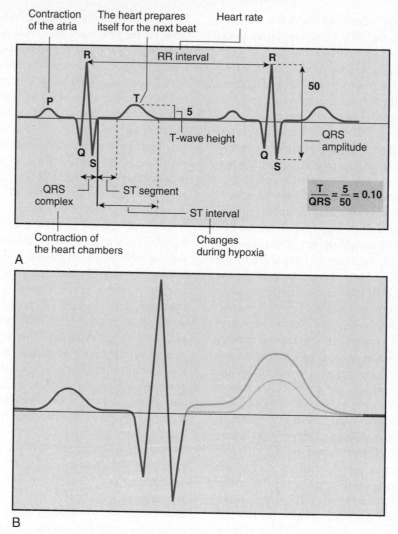

Fig. 15.1 ■ (A) Measurement of T/QRS ratio. (B) ST elevation and rise in the T wave.

The changes in the T/QRS ratio are highlighted as STAN events on the CTG trace if they are significant, and are recorded on a log event on the screen. The early studies in the 1980s showed promising results,[16,17] but inconsistent results from other studies[18] highlighted the need for computerization of ECG analysis and to take a rise in T/QRS from its own baseline levels instead of considering fixed values applicable to all fetuses. The ECG waveform analysis is used with the CTG (Table 15.1), as STAN or ST events can present owing to mechanical stresses

to the fetus or changes in the cardiac vector as the fetus descends in the birth canal.

The following guidelines apply for using the STAN technology.

This technology is applicable to fetuses who are 36 completed weeks' gestation or more. Significant ST events, when judged along with the CTG, indicate the need for intervention. This could be delivery of the fetus or alleviation of a cause of abnormal FHR changes such as oxytocin overstimulation or maternal hypotension. If the ST event occurred in the

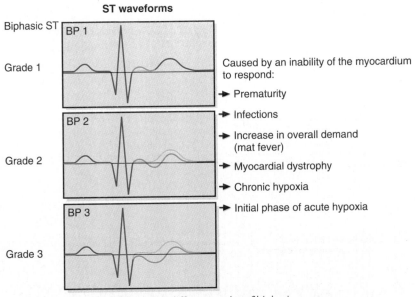

ST waveforms

Caused by an inability of the myocardium to respond:

→ Prematurity

→ Infections

→ Increase in overall demand (mat fever)

→ Myocardial dystrophy

→ Chronic hypoxia

→ Initial phase of acute hypoxia

Fig. 15.2 ■ The different grades of biphasic events.

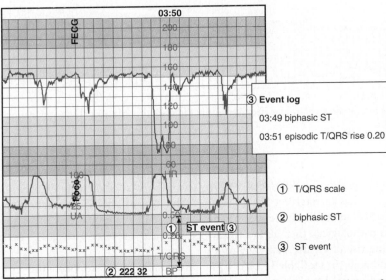

Fig. 15.3 ■ Recording of the fetal heart rate, contractions and computerized electrocardiograph waveform analysis of T/QRS plotted on the lower channel of the trace.

active phase of the second stage of labour, delivery within 20 min is recommended. In the second stage of labour, if the ST analyser was started when the CTG was normal, if the CTG trace became abnormal but there are no ST events, one could wait for 60 min before intervention. If significant ST events appear, then delivery should be carried out within 20 min.

When a STAN event is flagged up by the STAN equipment, one has to note the type of STAN event and the magnitude of change in that event (e.g., a baseline

TABLE 15.1			
Decision-Making Algorithm Using Computerised Analysis of ECG Waveform With Visual Interpretation of the CTG			
ST Analysis	**Intermediary CTG**	**Abnormal CTG**	**Preterminal CTG**
Episodic T/QRS rise	>0.15	>0.10	Immediate
Baseline T/QRS rise	>0.10	>0.05	Delivery
Biphasic ST	Continuous >5 min or >2 episodes of coupled biphasic 2 or biphasic 3	Continuous >2 min or >1 episode of coupled biphasic 2 or biphasic 3	

CTG, Cardiotocograph; *ECG*, electrocardiograph.

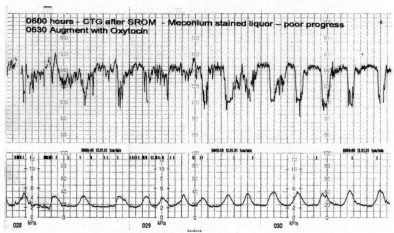

Fig. 15.4 ■ Cardiotocograph showing variable decelerations in early labour – related to hyperstimulation with oxytocin used for augmentation of labour.

T/QRS rise of >0.05 or episodic T/QRS rise of >0.10). Having noted this, one has to interpret the CTG as abnormal or intermediary to decide on the action to be taken. If the CTG is pathological, then action is warranted with a baseline rise of greater than 0.05 or an episodic rise greater than 0.10 (see Table 15.1).

The CTG classification used for STAN analysis[19] is slightly different from that used in the NICE guidelines.[20] A baseline rate of 110–150 bpm is considered normal, early and simple variable decelerations less than 60 beats and lasting less than 60 seconds (s) are considered normal, and variable decelerations less than 60 s but with beat loss greater than 60 beats are considered intermediary or suspicious.[19]

The case shown in Figures 15.4–15.6 illustrates the use of the STAN technology. A primigravida needed augmentation of labour with oxytocin because of poor progress. Variable decelerations are seen with oxytocin hyperstimulation. When oxytocin was stopped, the contractions became less frequent, lasting for a shorter duration and no progress was being made. The ST analyser was used for continuous additional information. Even if the fetus showed FHR decelerations and an increase in baseline rate, the absence of STAN events (significant ECG changes) would give the reassurance to continue with the oxytocin infusion with the aim of achieving a normal vaginal delivery.

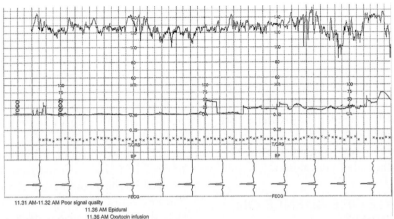

Fig. 15.5 ■ Oxytocin infusion was stopped. The cardiotocograph returned to normal and was reactive with no decelerations, but the contractions became less frequent. The ST analyser was connected and oxytocin infusion restarted.

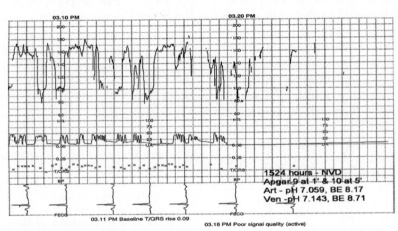

Fig. 15.6 ■ There was a gradual rise in the baseline rate following decelerations, followed by a reduction in baseline variability. No fetal blood sampling was done as there were no ST events. At 15.11 h there was an ST event of baseline rise indicating the need for delivery. A spontaneous delivery was imminent and the woman delivered spontaneously at 15.24 h. The baby had good Apgar scores and no evidence of metabolic acidosis.

STAN MONITORING AND NEW INTERNATIONAL FEDERATION OF OBSTETRICS AND GYNECOLOGY (FIGO) GUIDELINES ON CTG CLASSIFICATION

The STAN methodology was developed and validated using the first FIGO guidelines on CTG classification published in 1987. The resultant STAN guidelines on CTG interpretation were revised in 2007. However, a new FIGO classification system for CTG interpretation was introduced in 2015 and has raised the question whether the CTG interpretation arm of the STAN methodology is still valid if the new FIGO classification system is applied.[21] Investigators have mined and interrogated existing and large databases to identify CTG patterns, which are associated with ST events and adverse perinatal outcomes but are not covered by existing CTG classification and interpretation standards. The results show that CTG plus ST analysis may be undertaken, whatever the CTG classification system, provided a more physiologically based interpretation is deployed for CTG assessment in relation to ST events.[22] The revised STAN 2007 guidelines had a higher sensitivity for the detection of metabolic acidosis compared with the new FIGO 2015 guidelines for CTG classification (73% vs 43%, $P = .0002$).[23] Furthermore, it detected metabolic acidosis earlier with a mean time of 34 min than FIGO 2015 ($P = .002$).[23]

For these reasons we have continued to use STAN 2007 guidelines in the author's institution.

CURRENT STATE OF EVIDENCE ON STAN MONITORING

Several meta-analyses on the role of STAN monitoring have been published, albeit with variable selection criteria, inclusion or not, of revised data from primary trials, end points including caesarean delivery, metabolic acidosis, neonatal encephalopathy or death, low Apgar score and intubation for ventilation support.[24-27] The results have been inconsistent. Blix et al. used corrected datasets, the most appropriate methodology and analyses and concluded that CTG plus ST monitoring reduced operative vaginal delivery rates by 8% (RR, 0.92; 95% CI, 0.–0.99) and metabolic acidosis rates by 36% (OR, 0.64, 95% CI, 0.46–0.88).[26] This is in contrast with the nonsignificant reductions in metabolic acidosis reported in the Cochrane database of systematic reviews and meta-analyses, 28% (RR, 0.72, 95% CI, 0.43–1.20). [24]

CONCLUSION

Maternity units considering the introduction of the STAN methodology for intrapartum fetal surveillance should invest in intensive and mandatory staff training and retraining, particularly in fetal and labour physiology to achieve good outcome. Central monitoring systems and data archiving systems incorporated with the STAN systems assist in real time learning, case reviews and regular audits by analysis of data that improve performance. Audits indicate that poor perinatal outcomes with STAN are attributable to 'human factors' than poor technology.[28] No technology is 100% specific, and rarely a normal CTG could progress to a preterminal trace without ECG changes. Knowing

that there is higher risk of fetal acidosis when there is reduced or absent FHR variability with repeated decelerations in the CTG.[29,30] The STAN guidelines recommend intervention if the CTG shows repeated late or atypical variable decelerations for 1 hour (h) in a trace with absent variability[31]; Cochrane meta-analysis on ECG waveform analysis[24] in labour concludes that ST segment analysis reduces FBS rates (RR 0.61, 95% CI 0.41–0.91) and operative vaginal deliveries (RR 0.92, 95% CI 0.86–0.99) and mentions the use of scalp electrodes for ST waveform analysis. ST waveform analysis need not be a routine and can be selectively used on those with CTG using external means should they start showing a suspicious or abnormal CTG. NICE considered available studies on the use of STAN technology including cost effectiveness and came to the conclusion that neither it would recommend or not recommend the use of the STAN technology, thus allowing the units to decide on their preference.[32] The units that use this technology could use it appropriately (i.e., when the CTG is abnormal on an external trace) with the aim of reducing FBS and instrumental vaginal delivery rates.

REFERENCES

1. Hagberg B, Hagberg G, Beckung E, et al. Changing panorama of cerebral palsy in Sweden. VIII. Prevalence and origin in the birth year period 1991–1994. Acta Paediatr 2001;90:271–7.
2. Meberg A, Broch H. Etiology of cerebral palsy. J Perinat Med 2004;32:434–9.
3. Royal College of Obstetricians and Gynaecologists (RCOG). Each baby counts: key messages from 2015. London: RCOG; 2016. Online. Available: https://www.rcog.org.uk/globalassets/documents/guidelines/research-audit/rcog-each-baby-counts-report. [accessed 10.08.16].
4. NHS England. Saving babies' lives. A care bundle for reducing stillbirth. London: NHS; 2016. Online. Available: https://www.england.nhs.uk/wp-content/uploads/2016/03/saving-babies-lives-car-bundl. [accessed 10.08.16].
5. Ugwumadu A, Steer P, Parer B, et al. Time to optimise and enforce training in interpretation of intrapartum cardiotocograph. BJOG 2016;123(6):866–9.
6. Lear CL, Wassink G, Westgate JA, et al. The peripheral chemoreflex: indefatigable guardian of fetal physiological adaptation to labour. J Physiol 2018;596(23):5611–23.
7. Beard RW, Filshie GM, Knight CA, et al. The significance of the changes in the continuous fetal heart rate in the first stage of labour. J Obstet Gynaecol Br Commonw 1971;78:865–81.
8. Fleischer A, Schulman H, Jagani N, et al. The development of fetal acidosis in the presence of an abnormal fetal heart rate

tracing. I. The average for gestation age fetus. Am J Obstet Gynecol 1982;144:55–60.

9. Gillmer MDG, Combe D. Intrapartum fetal monitoring practice in the United Kingdom. Br J Obstet Gynaecol 1979;86:753–8.

10. Wheble AM, Gillmer MDG, Spencer JAD, et al. Changes in fetal monitoring practice in the UK: 1977–1984. Br J Obstet Gynaecol 1989;96:1140–7.

11. Sameshima H, Ikenoue T, Ikeda T, et al. Association of nonreassuring fetal heart rate patterns and subsequent cerebral palsy in pregnancies with intrauterine bacterial infection. Am J Perinatol 2005;22:181–7.

12. Maberry MC, Ramin SM, Gilstrap LC, et al. Intrapartum asphyxia in pregnancies complicated by intra-amniotic infection. Obstet Gynecol 1990;76(3 Pt 1):351–4.

13. Westgate J, Greene KR. How well is fetal blood sampling used in clinical practice? Br J Obstet Gynaecol 1999;106:774–82.

14. Rosen KG, Dagbjartsson A, Henriksson BA, et al. The relationship between circulating catecholamine and ST waveform in the fetal lamb electrocardiogram during hypoxia. Am J Obstet Gynecol 1984;149:190–5.

15. Amer-Wahlin I, Yli B, Arulkumaran S. Foetal ECG and STAN technology – a review. Eur Clinics Obstet Gynaecol 2005;1:61–73.

16. Lilja H, Arulkumaran S, Lindecrantz K, et al. Fetal ECG during labour: a presentation of a microprocessor system. J Biomed Eng 1988;10:348–50.

17. Arulkumaran S, Lilja H, Lindecrantz K, et al. Fetal ECG waveform analysis should improve fetal surveillance in labour. J Perinat Med 1990;187:13–22.

18. MacLachlan NA, Harding K, Spencer JAD, et al. Fetal heart rate, fetal acidaemia and the T/QRS ratio of the fetal ECG in labour. Br J Obstet Gynaecol 1991;99:26–31.

19. Amer-Wahlin I, Hellsten C, Noren H, et al. Cardiotocography only versus ST analysis of fetal electrocardiogram for intrapartum monitoring: a Swedish randomised controlled trial. Lancet 2001;358(9281):534–8.

20. National Institute for Health and Care Excellence (NICE). Intrapartum care for healthy women and their babies. NICE clinical guideline 190; 3 December 2014. Online. Available: https://www.nice.org.uk/guidance/cg190/resources/intrapartum-care-for-healthy-women-and-babies-35109866447557. [accessed 10.08.16].

21. Visser GH, Ayres-de-Campos D. FIGO consensus guidelines on intrapartum fetal monitoring: adjunctive technologies. Int J Gynaecol Obstet 2015;131:25–9.

22. Rosén KG, Norén H, Carlsson A. FHR patterns that become significant in connection with ST waveform changes and metabolic acidosis at birth. J Matern Fetal Neonatal Med. 2019 Oct;32(19):3288–3293.

23. Olofsson P, Norén H, Carlsson A. New FIGO and Swedish intrapartum cardiotocography classification systems incorporated in the fetal ECG ST analysis (STAN) interpretation algorithm: agreements and discrepancies in cardiotocography classification and evaluation of significant ST events. Acta Obstet Gynecol Scand 2018;97(2):219–28.

24. Neilson JP. Fetal electrocardiogram (ECG) for fetal monitoring during labour. Cochrane Database Syst Rev 2015;12:CD000116. [accessed 03.08.2022].

25. Saccone G, Schuit E, Amer-Wåhlin I, et al. Electrocardiogram ST analysis during labor: a systematic review and meta-analysis of randomized controlled trials. Obstet Gynecol 2016;127:127–35.

26. Blix E, Brurberg KG, Reierth E, et al. ST waveform analysis versus cardiotocography alone for intrapartum fetal monitoring: a systematic review and meta-analysis of randomized trials. Acta Obstet Gynecol Scand 2016;95:16–27.

27. Wetterslev J, Jakobsen JC, Gluud C. Trial sequential analysis in systematic reviews with meta-analysis. BMC Med Res Methodol 2017;17:39.

28. Doria V, Papageorghiou AT, Gustaffson A, et al. Review of the first 1502 cases of ECG–ST waveform analysis during labour in a teaching hospital. BJOG 2007;114(10):1202–7.

29. Williams KP, Galerneau F. Intrapartum fetal heart rate patterns in the prediction of neonatal acidemia. Am J Obstet Gynecol 2003;188:820–3.

30. Gull I, Jaffa AJ, Oren M, et al. Acid accumulation during end-stage bradycardia in term fetuses: how long is too long? Br J Obstet Gynaecol 1996;103:1096–101.

31. Amer-Wahlin I, Arulkumaran S, Hagberg H, et al. Fetal electrocardiogram: ST waveform analysis in intrapartum surveillance. BJOG 2007;114(10):1191–3.

32. National Institute for Health and care excellence. Final version of Addendum to intrapartum care: care for healthy women and babies. Clinical Guideline 190.1 Methods, evidence and recommendations -February 2017. Developed by the National Guideline Alliance, hosted by the Royal College of Obstetricians and Gynaecologists. https://www.nice.org.uk/guidance/cg190/evidence/addendum-190.1-pdf-4365472285. [accessed 03.08.2022].

16

MEDICOLEGAL ISSUES WITH CARDIOTOCOGRAPH AND CURRENT STRATEGIES TO REDUCE LITIGATION

PHILIP J. STEER

SHOULD WE BE USING CONTINUOUS ELECTRONIC MONITORING OF FETAL HEART RATE AND UTERINE CONTRACTIONS DURING LABOUR?

Electronic fetal monitoring (EFM), consisting of continuous recording of the fetal heart rate and uterine contractions (cardiotocograph, CTG), was first widely introduced in the 1960s. Already by 1970, an article in the *Nursing Mirror and Midwives Journal*[1] suggested that 'By means of electronic techniques it is now possible with a minimum of staff to obtain continuous and reliable information on the intrauterine pressure and the fetal heart rate during labour. We have reason to believe that these measures will greatly diminish the risk of hypoxic fetal brain damage during labour'. By the end of the 1970s, in the majority of maternity units in the United Kingdom, at least a third of labours were being monitored by CTG and in a few units it had already become universal.[2] However, when it became apparent that national rates of cerebral palsy were not falling, doubts began to creep in, and these were increased following the publication of the Dublin randomized controlled trial in 1985, which showed no clear evidence of benefit of CTG over intermittent auscultation.[3] In 1986 in the *British Medical Journal*,[4] Prof Peter Howie wrote in relation to CTG that 'its use has been the subject of deep controversy ... regular intermittent auscultation may prove to be sufficient in low risk mothers'. The controversy deepened when the follow-up to the Dublin trial showed no reduction in cerebral palsy rates in the EFM group.[5] However,

a case–control study by Gaffney et al. of intrapartum care, cerebral palsy and perinatal death, published in 1994, reported that the fetal heart rate pattern was abnormal in 67% of labours ending in perinatal death, and in 23% of labours with subsequent cerebral palsy, compared with only 10% in controls.[6] This confirmed that there was a link between an abnormal fetal heart rate pattern and a poor outcome for the baby, both short term and long term. In 1995, two influential meta-analyses were published. The first, by Vintzileos et al.,[7] of nine trials reported that, although there was no overall reduction in perinatal mortality from the use of CTG monitoring, hypoxic deaths were reduced by almost 60%. The second, by Thacker et al.,[8] of 12 trials reported a statistically significant 50% decrease in the incidence of neonatal seizures. These data have been sufficient to ensure that EFM continues to be the standard of care for intrapartum surveillance, and in developed countries it is considered mandatory in high-risk labours.[9]

THE INCIDENCE OF SUBSTANDARD CARE AS A CONTRIBUTOR TO POOR OUTCOME

The study by Gaffney et al.[6] went further than simply analysing the proportion of abnormal fetal heart rate patterns in relation to outcome and assessed the proportion of cases where there was a 'failure to respond to signs of fetal distress'. In cases of perinatal death, this was 50%, and in cases of cerebral palsy, 26%, compared with only 7% in cases with a normal outcome. Extrapolation of their regional data to the whole of the UK suggested that, in any given year, cerebral palsy associated with a failure to respond to evidence of fetal compromise would occur in 174 cases. Even if only half of such cases lead to successful litigation, the cost of monitoring failure becomes enormous because of the very large monetary value of individual settlements. The findings of Gaffney et al. amplified those of a 1990 publication of a review of 64 cases with a poor outcome from the records of the Medical Protection Society.[10] They found that, in 11 cases, CTG monitoring had not been carried out when it should have been and was technically unsatisfactory in a further 6 (27% overall), and the CTG trace was physically missing in 19 (30%). However, CTG abnormalities were either not recognized or ignored in 14 cases (22%), and in only 14 cases (22%) was the abnormality noted and responded to appropriately. A further study by the same authors, of 41 cases from the records of the Association for the Victims of Medical Accidents (AVMA), concluded that 'inadequate fetal monitoring and insufficient supervision of junior doctors were implicated in a high proportion of accidents, some junior doctors and midwives cannot recognize abnormal CTG traces, and most receive inadequate training in CTG monitoring'.[11] Such was the concern about preventable injury to the fetus during labour that the UK government funded a national Confidential Enquiry into Stillbirths and Deaths in Infancy (CESDI). The sixth annual report, of births in the year 1st January to 31st December 1997 and published in 1999,[12] detailed a study of 567 cases of poor outcome. Entirely appropriate care was found in only 28%. In a further 21%, substandard care was identified but proper care would not have changed the outcome. Worryingly, substandard care that could possibly have affected the outcome was identified in 28%, and the substandard care was likely to have affected the outcome in a further 22%. Therefore, in fully half of cases, the outcome might have been changed by correct management. The authors of the report commented that 'fetal surveillance problems were the commonest cause (of problems in labour), with CTG interpretation ... the most frequent criticism'. A report by the National Health Service Litigation Authority (NHSLA, renamed National Health Service (NHS) Resolution in 2017) in 2009 of a study of 100 stillbirth claims, reported that misinterpretation of the CTG occurred in 34 cases,[13] involving midwives

in 25 cases, registrars in 8 and consultants in only 4, highlighting the inadequate supervision of junior staff.

From 2015 onward, the Royal College of Obstetricians and Gynaecologists (RCOG) carried out an annual audit of births in the UK. Their first full report, of births in 2015, detailed adverse outcome in 1136 cases, with 126 intrapartum stillbirths, 156 neonatal deaths and 854 cases of severe brain injury (with the associated risk of long-term cerebral palsy).[14] Worryingly, in the 727 adequate quality case reviews analysed, there was substandard care reported in 552 – 76%. In the subsequent annual audits, these figures did not improve significantly, so that by 2018 there were still 1145 adverse outcomes with 859 cases of severe brain injury and substandard care in 74%.[14] The 2015 report highlighted a failure to take into account additional risk factors – reduced fetal movements, fetal growth restriction, meconium staining of the amniotic fluid, suspected infection (pyrexia), intrapartum haemorrhage, prolonged labour (associated with the use of syntocinon for augmentation) and previous caesarean section (CS) – when assessing the significance of CTG abnormalities. This theme was addressed in more detail in subsequent reports, highlighting loss of situational awareness (e.g., overemphasis on the significance of the CTG, ignoring the additional risk factors), lack of team working, inadequate training and avoidable delays in delivering the baby once impending compromise had been identified (2017 audit report).

THE MEDICOLEGAL CRISIS

Before the 1980s, litigation against doctors alleging malpractice was rare. When I first qualified in 1971, my annual subscription to the Medical Defence Union was £5 for a year's cover. However, this started to rise in the 1980s, and by 1987 it had risen to more than £300 per annum. Over the next 3 years, the steady rise of the previous 15 years changed to an acceleration, so that by 1990 my annual subscription was £1400. As a consequence of the resulting erosion of annual salaries, especially in high-risk specialties such as obstetrics, health authorities in 1990 took over financial responsibility for negligence attributable to medical and dental staff employed in the NHS. In 1995, the NHSLA was set up to administer a

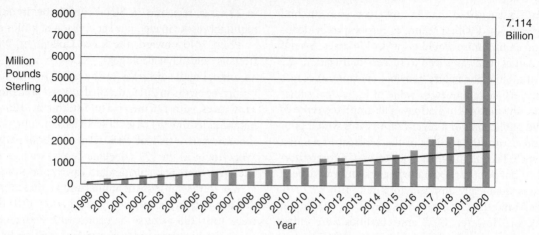

Fig. 16.1 ■ Annual value of clinical negligence claims to the National Health Service (*NHS*) Litigation Authority – NHS Resolution-up to and including 2020–21. (The data have been extracted from the annual reports of the NHS litigation Authority/ NHS Resolution. The latest report is at https://resolution.nhs.uk/corporate-reports/)

national scheme of indemnity for medical and associated staffs. They set up a system called the 'Clinical Negligence Scheme for Trusts' (CNST), which linked the cover premiums charged to individual care groups (e.g. Hospital Trusts) to the development of good clinical care guidelines within the Trust. It then became apparent that good-quality guidelines had no discernible impact on the rate of medical legal claims, and in 2014 the CNST system was abandoned in favour of premiums based on the historical rate of claims attributed to each individual Trust. The NHSLA has published its annual accounts since 1998, and these show that, from an annual pay-out of £70 million in 1998, the amounts paid out have risen dramatically (Fig. 16.1), so that in the financial year 2020–2021 £7.114 billion was disbursed to claimants and their lawyers. The 2020–2021 accounts show that obstetrics accounted for 11% of all clinical negligence claims received in that financial year; this proportion rose to 59% when the value of the claims was considered rather than their number (Fig. 16.2).[15]

Settlements for individual claims have now reached £37 million.[16] The dramatic increase in the cost of settlements from 2017 was the result of changes to the Ogden formula, the interest rate used to calculate payouts.[17] Until then, it was assumed that lump sum payments accrued interest at the rate of 2.5%, but due to low inflation following the worldwide financial crash of 2018, this was reduced

to −0.75% in March 2017 and raised to −0.25% in 2019. This resulted in an overnight 2.5-fold increase in the size of compensation payments for injury due to negligence. The 2020–2021 NHS Resolution report records that claims received are now running at an average of £6887 per birth (Fig. 16.3), with actual payments for historical claims averaging £1533 per birth – £9.2 million pounds annually for a maternity unit delivering 6000 babies per year.

TRAINING IN CARDIOTOCOGRAPH INTERPRETATION

Despite the acknowledged importance of correct CTG interpretation during labour, policies to improve performance remain in their infancy. In 2001, Young et al.[18] reported that 74% of low Apgar scores at the North Staffs hospital in the UK were associated with suboptimal care. They introduced regular low-Apgar feedback meetings involving labour ward staff and found that the incidence of suboptimal care dropped to 23%. However, with time the proportion of suboptimal care increased again to 32%, at which point they made CTG training compulsory for labour ward staff. The subsequent rate of suboptimal care fell to 9%. In most occupations, compulsory training for a key activity would not be seen as revolutionary; however, even in developed countries, most CTG training is based

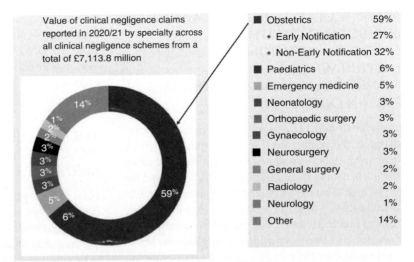

Value of clinical negligence claims reported in 2020/21 by specialty across all clinical negligence schemes from a total of £7,113.8 million

Obstetrics	59%
• Early Notification	27%
• Non-Early Notification	32%
Paediatrics	6%
Emergency medicine	5%
Neonatology	3%
Orthopaedic surgery	3%
Gynaecology	3%
Neurosurgery	3%
General surgery	2%
Radiology	2%
Neurology	1%
Other	14%

Fig. 16.2 ■ Value of clinical negligence claims reported in 2020-2021 by specialty. NHS Resoltion.

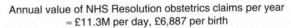

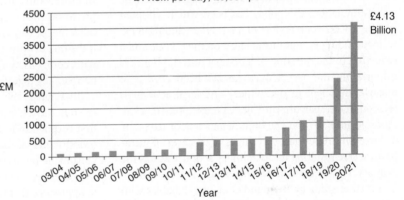

Annual value of NHS Resolution obstetrics claims per year ≈ £11.3M per day, £6,887 per birth

Fig. 16.3 ■ Annual obstetric claims per year from 2003–2004 to 2020–21.

around a few formal lectures, self-directed learning and ad hoc mentoring. In the NHS, CTG courses are rarely run as part of the maternity unit official training programme, instead being provided by charities such as Baby Lifeline.[19] Web-based electronic systems for training are available, provided for example by K2 medical systems[20] and the RCOG.[21] However, such systems are not based upon assessment of individual requirements, nor are the self-assessment components monitored by the supervising authorities in the NHS. It is a crucial weakness of the system that in most maternity units there is no systematic assessment of birth attendants' ability to interpret CTGs. This contrasts with the situation in, for

example, aviation – where pilots' abilities are tested formally on a 6-monthly basis. Anyone who fails the assessment is taken out of service and retrained until they reach the appropriate standard (which is, for example, 100% success at taking off and landing without error or mishap). In one detailed study of the benefits of a computer-assisted teaching programme for intrapartum fetal monitoring, the success rate of medical staff in the interpretation of CTGs rose from about 70% before training to about 85% afterward; however, 100% correct interpretation remained elusive. Worryingly, the success rate of midwives was originally about 50% but rose to only about 70% after training.[22]

A PARTICULAR MEDICOLEGAL RISK IS ASSOCIATED WITH THE USE OF OXYTOCIN INFUSION TO AUGMENT LABOUR WHEN THE CTG IS NONREASSURING OR ABNORMAL/ PATHOLOGICAL.

In the 1960s and 1970s, Kieran O'Driscoll, Master (in charge of the labour ward) at the National Maternity Hospital in Dublin, promoted a concept that he dubbed 'the active management of labour',[23] which required the use of high-dose oxytocin infusion in more than 50% of nulliparous women in labour.[24,25] He subsequently claimed that in his unit it was preventing the rise in CS rates that have been seen widely throughout the developed world over the past 50 years.[26] Despite editorials in the *British Medical Journal*[27,28] and the *British Journal of Obstetrics and Gynaecology*[29] warning against the use of active management because of the dangers of uterine hyperstimulation, the policy has been widely adopted despite a Cochrane review of 14 trials including 8033 women finding no significant effect on the CS rate and a reduction in the duration of labour of only 1.3 hours.[30] Importantly, the use of oxytocin has been cited as a major component in disciplinary and legal actions in relation to intrapartum care. For example, Jonsson et al. reported in 2007 that the 'injudicious use of oxytocin' occurred in more than two thirds of 60 cases of intrapartum care resulting in disciplinary action and was the primary reason for disciplinary action in one third.[31] In a further study by Berglund et al. of 177 babies with severe birth asphyxia due to malpractice/poor supervision, the incautious use of oxytocin was implicated in 71%.[32] The latest recommendations of the National Institute for Health and Care Excellence (NICE) in the United Kingdom[9] now state (recommendation 1.12.10) 'do not routinely offer the package known as active management of labour', and (recommendation 1.12.18) 'for all women with confirmed delay in the established first stage of labour: explain to her that using oxytocin after spontaneous or artificial rupture of the membranes will bring forward the time of birth but will not influence the mode of birth or other outcomes'. They highlight that, if the CTG is not entirely normal, then any oxytocin infusion should be reduced or stopped and/or a tocolytic drug offered (a suggested regimen is subcutaneous terbutaline 0.25 mg). A 2015 meta-analysis reported that discontinuing oxytocin after the active phase of labour is established significantly decreases rates of CS (OR 0.51, 95% CI 0.35, 0.74) as well as those of uterine hyperstimulation (OR 0.33, 95% CI 0.19, 0.58),[33] so there seems every reason to limit the use of oxytocin as far as possible, for both clinical and medicolegal reasons.

THE PRINCIPLES OF LEGAL PRACTICE AS APPLIED TO MEDICINE

For a medical practitioner to be found guilty of medical negligence, two aspects of each case have to be considered separately. Firstly, was there a breach of duty? Every doctor has a duty of care to their patient that requires them to treat the patient according to the accepted standards of the time. Did the doctor's practice meet those accepted standards? Secondly, causation needs to be established. In other words, was there a direct link between the failure to practice according to accepted standards and the outcome for which compensation is being claimed? Even if the doctor's practice fell well below an acceptable standard, compensation will not be paid if there is no clear link between the unacceptable care and an adverse outcome.

In English law, negligence was initially defined by reference to a hypothetical reasonable person, a concept first codified in Roman law as the 'bonus paterfamilias' (good father of the family). In Victorian times, such a reasonable but average person was sometimes referred to as the 'man on the Clapham omnibus'. It is important to appreciate that the standards applied in clinical practice are those of the average clinician appropriate for the task, and not those of the super specialist. Acceptable practice is commonly a range of options rather than a single policy, which is why it is so hard to write general guidelines. The grounds by which breach of duty should be judged were particularly well defined in the 1957 case of *Bolam* v. *Friern Hospital Management Committee*.[34] This related to a patient suffering from a mental illness who sustained a fracture during the use of electroconvulsive therapy. There were, according to expert witnesses, two conflicting bodies of medical opinion, one of which favoured the routine use of muscle-relaxant drugs to prevent fracture, whereas the other felt that the risk from the relaxant itself was too high for routine use so that it should be used only when there were specific indications. The judge directed the jury as follows:

A doctor is not negligent, if he is acting in accordance with a practice accepted as proper by a responsible body of medical men skilled in that particular art, merely because there is a body of such opinion that takes a contrary view.

In other words, as long as a reasonable number of doctors would do what you did in a particular circumstance, your actions are not negligent.

A particularly important obstetric case occurred in 1981, that of *Whitehouse* v. *Jordan*.[35] This related to the attempted delivery of a baby who had sustained 'brain damage'. Following a prolonged labour, the obstetrician conducted a trial of forceps delivery, but after six pulls there was no movement and so he abandoned the procedure and performed a CS. It was alleged that he was negligent because he had considered that forceps could be used to deliver the baby when in fact the outcome showed that this was not possible. Although the primary court held the obstetrician to be negligent, this decision was reversed by the Court of Appeal and the reversal was confirmed by the House of Lords (which has since become the UK Supreme Court). They concluded that 'an error of clinical judgment by a doctor is not the same thing as negligence. The test of an error of judgment in such a case is the standard of care of the ordinary skilled man exercising and professing to have a particular skill. Accordingly an error of judgment might or might not have been negligent'. The obstetrician, Mr Joe Jordan, was found not guilty of negligence. What this means is that, although a course of action might be seen to have been unequivocally wrong in retrospect (in this case the baby would probably have survived intact if the caesarean had been done without a trial of forceps), it can often be an acceptable (and even the most appropriate) action when carried out without knowledge of the eventual outcome. Medical practitioners are not expected to be able to foresee the future, only to take reasonable action.

Another legal landmark occurred in 1997, with the case of *Bolitho* v. *City and Hackney Health Authority*.[36] This again was not an obstetric case but related to a 2-year-old boy with a past history of hospital treatment for croup. Following admission to hospital, he had difficulty in breathing and turned white on two occasions; unfortunately, the two doctors who were called failed to attend (although they could have done

if they had made it an appropriate priority). Following apparent recovery, the boy later suffered total respiratory failure and cardiac arrest resulting in severe brain damage, and he subsequently died. Although the lower court and the Court of Appeal decided that because a responsible body of professional opinion 'espoused by distinguished and truthful experts' held that even if they had attended, they would not necessarily have intubated the child and thereby prevented the cardiac arrest, the House of Lords held that a doctor could be held liable for negligence 'despite a body of professional opinion sanctioning his conduct where it had not been demonstrated to the judges' satisfaction that the body of opinion relied on was reasonable or responsible'. They went on to say that 'if it could be demonstrated that professional opinion was not capable of withstanding logical analysis, the judge was entitled to hold that the body of opinion was not reasonable or responsible'. However, in the case of Bolitho, the Court held that the body of opinion was in fact reasonable and therefore there was, in this particular case, no evidence of negligence. Nonetheless, the Court had established that not only must a course of action be that which would be supported by a reasonable body of medical opinion, but it must also stand up to logical analysis. You cannot escape liability for doing something unreasonable just because others would do the same.

The most important recent case is probably that of *Montgomery* v. *Lanarkshire Health Board (Scotland)*, 2015 SC 11.[37] This was again an obstetric case. Nadine Montgomery was a diabetic woman of short stature, and her first baby was predicted by ultrasound to weigh more than 4 kg. She was not offered a CS, but instead labour was induced. She was not told about the potential risk of shoulder dystocia, and when this occurred the baby experienced severe asphyxia and later developed cerebral palsy. Although two lower courts rejected a claim of negligence, accepting that many obstetricians would also have encouraged vaginal birth, the UK Supreme Court upheld an appeal in favour of the claimant, affirming that women have a right to be told about any material risks in order to make an autonomous decision about how they wished to give birth. The level of risk to be disclosed is not judged on what the doctors think is important but instead on the importance attached to it by the patient. Thus obstetricians who do not advise their patients of all material risks (whether important because they are common or because they are uncommon but particularly serious) are likely to be judged negligent. When there are options available, the patient should decide which they prefer, and not the doctor. If a caesarean is a reasonable option, even though it may not be preferable from a population point of view, women are entitled to choose it.

A procedural point is that it is the courts that decide negligence, and obstetric experts who give evidence should avoid making such judgements. Instead, their evidence should indicate whether the care delivered to the patient was of a proper professional standard, and if the care fell below this standard, then (in civil cases) whether on the balance of probability the deficiency in care led to the adverse outcome. 'On the balance of probability' means a likelihood of 51% or more. In recent years there has been increasing recourse to the use of the criminal law when the care has been particularly substandard. In such situations, obstetricians and midwives may be accused of manslaughter. This is quite difficult to define,[38] but essentially a judgement of manslaughter is likely to be made if the care given was reckless or so grossly deficient that the adverse outcome ought to have been foreseeable (the final judgement is usually made by a jury). Examples might include doctors who refuse to attend despite an obvious duty to do so, or who are intoxicated by alcohol or drugs or who act with a blatant disregard for the safety of the patient. In such cases, the criterion for a judgement of manslaughter to be made is much higher than in a civil case, being the criminal standard of 'beyond a reasonable doubt'.

THE WAY FORWARD

The previous account has highlighted the potential value of continuous intrapartum EFM. However, it has proven difficult to realize its full value in practice. Rates of cerebral palsy associated with intrapartum asphyxia have not shown any significant decline, while litigation rates alleging malpractice continue to increase. The proportion of legal cases involving misinterpretation of CTG traces has remained stubbornly high over the past three decades. Part of the problem in this regard is the constant turnover of staff, with experienced clinicians being promoted away from the labour ward and

replaced by less-experienced trainees. In an attempt to deal with this problem, several groups have developed a computerized approach to CTG interpretation. The Plymouth group, led by obstetrician Prof Keith Greene and bioengineer Robert Keith, first reported their system combining the use of neural networks with rule-based algorithms in 1994[39–41] and by 1995 published a study showing that the system could work as well as the best of 17 UK experts at the detection of pathological fetal heart rate patterns.[42] They subsequently set up a prospective randomized trial of the technology,[43] which took a long time to fund and carry out because of the very large numbers of participants expected to be needed to show an effect on significant outcomes such as perinatal mortality and hypoxic ischaemic encephalopathy. In the event, the trial (the INFANT trial) lasted for 5 years and included more than 46,000 births in 24 different maternity units.[44] Perhaps the most striking finding was that, in the total study group (which was relatively high risk because it included only women with an indication for EFM), there were only three intrapartum stillbirths (one per 15,347 births). This was much lower than predicted. For example in the CTG arm of the 1985 Dublin trial of CTG versus intermittent auscultation,[3] the rate of intrapartum stillbirth was 1 per 2617 births, and the national UK rate of intrapartum stillbirth in 2015 was almost three times higher at 1 in 5740 births.[14] A low rate of neonatal mortality was also found in the INFANT trial – 1 case per 4661 births, giving an overall perinatal mortality rate of 0.28 per 1000 (it was 2.14 per 1000 in the Dublin trial and 0.39 per 1000 in the UK in 2015). Perhaps what the INFANT study showed most strikingly is the protective power of being in a clinical trial, with all the heightened surveillance that this involves.

However, despite the overall low rate of perinatal mortality, it was found that in a sub-analysis of 71 cases of adverse outcome (intrapartum stillbirth, neonatal death and admission to special care with acidosis), 38% of these cases were associated with substandard care, which if it had been prevented would have likely have resulted in the baby surviving without injury (there was some degree of substandard care in 64% overall).[45] The substandard care was mainly failure to appreciate the importance of additional risk factors such as fetal growth restriction, meconium staining of the amniotic fluid, maternal pyrexia, prolonged labour, uterine hyperstimulation with oxytocin and delays in responding to a recognised CTG abnormality.

Another computerized approach has been developed by the Sis-Porto group (Ayres-de-Campos and colleagues) in Portugal.[46] As with the INFANT system, its complexity meant that it required 19 years to develop it. Called Ominview-Sis-Porto, an off-line analysis of its performance was comparable with that of three experienced clinicians, in terms of both classification of the fetal heart rate pattern[47] and prediction of newborn umbilical artery blood pH.[48] However, the developers have now performed a prospective randomized controlled trial similar to that of the INFANT system (although with much smaller numbers),[49] and the results showed that computerised interpretation made no significant difference to the outcome.

It would appear that part of the problem with CTG interpretation has been the emphasis on pattern recognition, without sufficient emphasis on the interpretation of heart rate changes in the context of fetal pathophysiology. Intrapartum factors such as the duration of labour, maternal (and therefore fetal) fever, infection, meconium staining of the amniotic fluid and mechanical forces/trauma play an equal (and sometimes more important) role in making a correct assessment of fetal condition and the need for expedited delivery. There needs to be an understanding that hypoxia/acidosis is the major causative factor in fewer than 50% of babies who are born in poor condition.[50] Training of intrapartum attendants in CTG interpretation and the management of labour is intermittent and fragmented and has no agreed curriculum, and effective training and assessment tools to determine the competence of individual practitioners need to be developed.[51] In 2019, the RCOG and the Royal College of Midwives set up a joint committee to look at ways of improving intrapartum care. They commissioned a pilot study of a system to incorporate routine assessment of risk factors alongside fetal heart rate monitoring, which demonstrated that an intrapartum score adding six additional risk factors (oxytocin infusion, uterine tachysystole, meconium staining of the amniotic fluid, maternal pyrexia, bleeding and suspected fetal growth restriction) to four FHR variables (baseline rate, variability, repetitive or prolonged decelerations) was able to predict adverse outcome with an area under the receiver operator curve of 0.85.[52] A similar approach is being developed under the direction of

The Healthcare Improvement Studies (THIS) Institute in Cambridge and funded by the UK Department of Health.[53] Time will tell if such a system can reduce the devastating effect of substandard care and the ensuing litigation on families and the maternity services.

REFERENCES

[1] Lundström P. Monitoring the foetus in utero. Nurs Mirror Midwives J 1970;130:20.

[2] Gillmer MD, Combe D. Intrapartum fetal monitoring practice in the United Kingdom. Br J Obstet Gynaecol 1979;86:760.

[3] MacDonald D, Grant A, Sheridan-Pereira M, et al. The Dublin randomized controlled trial of intrapartum fetal heart rate monitoring. Am J Obstet Gynecol 1985;152:524–39.

[4] Howie PW. Fetal monitoring in labour. Br Med J 1986;292:427–8.

[5] Grant A, O'Brien N, Joy MT, et al. Cerebral palsy among children born during the Dublin randomised trial of intrapartum monitoring. Lancet 1989;2:1233–6.

[6] Gaffney G, Sellers S, Flavell V, et al. Case-control study of intrapartum care, cerebral palsy, and perinatal death. Br Med J 1994;308:743–50.

[7] Vintzileos AM, Nochimson DJ, Guzman ER, et al. Intrapartum electronic fetal heart rate monitoring versus intermittent auscultation: a meta-analysis. Obstet Gynecol 1995;85:149–55.

[8] Thacker SB, Stroup DF, Peterson HB. Efficacy and safety of intrapartum electronic fetal monitoring: an update. Obstet Gynecol 1995;86:613–20.

[9] NICE. Intrapartum care: care of healthy women and their babies during childbirth. Clinical guideline 190 (updated 2017). 2014. Available: https://www.nice.org.uk/guidance/cg190. [accessed 29.10.2021].

[10] Ennis M, Vincent CA. Obstetric accidents: a review of 64 cases. Br Med J 1990;300:1365–7.

[11] Vincent CA, Martin T, Ennis M. Obstetric accidents: the patient's perspective. Br J Obstet Gynaecol 1991;98:390–5.

[12] Confidential inquiry into stillbirths and deaths in infancy: sixth annual report, 1st January to 31st December 1997. London: Maternal and child health research consortium; 1999.

[13] NHSLA. Study of stillbirth claims. 2009. Available from: NHS Resolution. https://resolution.nhs.uk/corporate-reports/.

[14] Each Baby Counts (repository of reports). Available: https://www.rcog.org.uk/en/guidelines-research-services/audit-quality-improvement/each-baby-counts/reports-updates/; [accessed 29.10.2021].

[15] NHS Resolution Annual Reports. Available: https://resolution.nhs.uk/corporate-reports/

[16] Devonshires Claims. Family awarded £37 million in the largest NHS maternity Negligence Claim. Available: https://devonshiresclaims.co.uk/family-awarded-37-million-in-the-largest-nhs-maternity-negligence-claim/; [accessed 29.10.2021].

[17] Ogden tables: actuarial compensation tables for injury and death. UK Gov. Available: https://www.gov.uk/government/

publications/ogden-tables-actuarial-compensation-tables-for-injury-and-death [accessed 29.10.2021].

[18] Young P, Hamilton R, Hodgett S, et al. Reducing risk by improving standards of intrapartum fetal care. J R Soc Med 2001;94:226–31.

[19] Baby Lifeline Training. Available: https://babylifelinetraining. org.uk/home/ [accessed 29.10.2021].

[20] K2MS Perinatal Training Programme (PTP). Available: https://www.k2ms.com/ptp/ [accessed 29.10.2021].

[21] RCOG CTG training. Available: https://www.e-lfh.org.uk/ programmes/electronic-fetal-monitoring/.

[22] Beckley S, Stenhouse E, Greene K. The development and evaluation of a computer-assisted teaching programme for intrapartum fetal monitoring. BJOG 2000;107:1138–44.

[23] O'Driscoll K, Meagher D. Active management of labour. London: Saunders; 1980.

[24] O'Driscoll K, Jackson RJA, Gallagher JT. Prevention of prolonged labour. Br Med J 1969;ii(5655):447–8.

[25] O'Driscoll K, Stronge JM, Minogue M. Active management of labour. Br Med J 1973;iii:135–7.

[26] O'Driscoll K, Foley M, MacDonald D. Active management of labour as an alternative to cesarean section for dystocia. Obstet Gynecol 1984;63:485–90.

[27] Thornton JG, Lilford RJ. Active management of labour: current knowledge and research issues [published erratum appears in BMJ 1994 Sep 17;309(6956): 704] [see comments]. Br Med J 1994;309:366–9.

[28] Thornton JG. Active management of labour. Br Med J 1996;313:378.

[29] Oláh KS, Gee H. The active mismanagement of labour. Br J Obstet Gynaecol 1996;103:729–31.

[30] Wei S, Wo BL, Qi HP, et al. Early amniotomy and early oxytocin for prevention of, or therapy for, delay in first stage spontaneous labour compared with routine care. Cochrane Database Syst Rev 2013;8:CD006794.

[31] Jonsson M, Nordén SL, Hanson U. Analysis of malpractice claims with a focus on oxytocin use in labour. Acta Obs Gynecol Scand 2007;86:315–9.

[32] Berglund S, Grunewald C, Pettersson H, et al. Severe asphyxia due to delivery-related malpractice in Sweden 1990–2005. BJOG 2008;115:316–23.

[33] Vlachos DEG, Pergialiotis V, Papantoniou N, et al. Oxytocin discontinuation after the active phase of labor is established. J Matern Fetal Neonatal Med 2015;28:1421–7.

[34] McNair J. Bolam v Friern hospital management committee – [1957] 2 all ER 118. All Engl. Law Rep. 1957;2.

[35] HL. Whitehouse vs Jordan [_1981] 1 all ER 267, _[1981] 1 WLR 246, 125 Sol Jo 167. 1981.

[36] Bolitho v city and Hackney health authority. 1997. https:// publications.parliament.uk/pa/ld199798/ldjudgmt/jd971113/ boli01.htm

[37] Montgomery v Lanarksh. Heal. Board [2015]UKSC 11). Montgomery (Appellant) v Lanarkshire health board (respondent) (Scotland) [2015] UKSC 11). 2015. Available: https//www.supremecourt.uk/decided-cases/docs/ UKSC_2013_0136_Judgment.pdf.

[38] Crown Prosecution Service (UK) Homicide – murder and manslaughter. Available: https://www.cps.gov.uk/legal-

guidance/homicide-murder-and-manslaughter [accessed 29.10.2021].

[39] Keith RD, Westgate J, Ifeachor EC, et al. Suitability of artificial neural networks for feature extraction from cardiotocogram during labour. Med Biol Eng Comput 1994;32:S51–7.

[40] Keith RD, Greene KR. Development, evaluation and validation of an intelligent system for the management of labour. [Review] [29 refs]. Baillieres Clin Obstet Gynaecol 1994;8:583–605.

[41] Keith RD, Westgate J, Hughes GW, et al. Preliminary evaluation of an intelligent system for the management of labour. J Perinat Med 1994;22:345–50.

[42] Keith RD, Beckley S, Garibaldi JM, et al. A multicentre comparative study of 17 experts and an intelligent computer system for managing labour using the cardiotocogram. Br J Obstet Gynaecol 1995;102:688–700.

[43] Brocklehurst P, Group TIC. A study of an intelligent system to support decision making in the management of labour using the cardiotocograph – the INFANT study protocol. BMC Pregnancy Childbirth 2016;16:10.

[44] Brocklehurst P, Field DJ, Juszczak E, et al. The INFANT trial. Lancet 2017;390. Available: https://doi.org/10.1016/S0140-6736(17)31594-5.

[45] Steer PJ, Kovar I, McKenzie C, et al. Computerised analysis of intrapartum fetal heart rate patterns and adverse outcomes in the INFANT trial. BJOG 2019;126:1354–61.

[46] Ayres-de-Campos D, Sousa P, Costa A, et al. Omniview-SisPorto 3.5 – a central fetal monitoring station with online alerts based on computerized cardiotocogram+ST event analysis. J Perinat Med 2008;36:260–4.

[47] Costa MA, Ayres-de-Campos D, Machado AP, et al. Comparison of a computer system evaluation of intrapartum cardiotocographic events and a consensus of clinicians. J Perinat Med 2010;38:191–5.

[48] Costa A, Santos C, Ayres-de-Campos D, et al. Access to computerised analysis of intrapartum cardiotocographs improves clinicians' prediction of newborn umbilical artery blood pH. BJOG 2010;117:1288–93.

[49] Nunes I, Ayres-de-Campos D, Ugwumadu A, et al. Central fetal monitoring with and without computer analysis: a randomized controlled trial. Obstet Gynecol 2017;129:83–90.

[50] Lissauer TJ, Steer PJ. The relation between the need for intubation at birth, abnormal cardiotocograms in labour and cord artery blood gas and pH values. Br J Obstet Gynaecol 1986;93:1060–6.

[51] Ugwumadu A, Steer P, Parer B, et al. Time to optimise and enforce training in interpretation of intrapartum cardiotocograph. BJOG An Int J Obstet Gynaecol 2016;123:866–9. Available: https://doi.org/10.1111/1471-0528.13846.

[52] Steer PJ, Yau CWH, Blott M, Lattey K, Nwandison M, Uddin Z, Winter C, Draycott T. A case-control study of the interaction of fetal heart rate abnormalities, fetal growth restriction, meconium in the amniotic fluid and tachysystole, in relation to the outcome of labour. BJOG. 2022 Sep 27. doi: 10.1111/1471-0528.17302. Online ahead of print.

[53] THIS. Avoiding Brain Injury in Childbirth. Available: https:// www.thiscovery.org/project/abc [accessed 29.10.2021].

17

FETAL WELLBEING IN LABOUR – NATIONAL INITIATIVES, CHALLENGES AND THE FUTURE

LOUISE DEWICK ■ RACHNA BAHL ■ WENDY RANDALL ■ TIM DRAYCOTT

THE NATIONAL AMBITION

The national maternity ambition, launched in November 2015 by the UK Department of Health, aimed to halve the number of stillbirths, intrapartum brain injuries and neonatal and maternal deaths in England by 2030 so that England would be one of the safest places in the world to have a baby. This was also part of the wider patient-safety strategy to reduce avoidable harm in the NHS by 50%[1] and in 2017, a National Maternity Safety Strategy was launched with an accelerated ambition to achieve these improvements by 2025.[2]

Assessment of fetal heart rate patterns is currently one of the main methods to assess fetal well-being both antenatally and intrapartum. Accurate, consistent interpretation and action on fetal heart rate patterns has been identified as an important strategy to reduce adverse outcomes. The Kirkup report published in 2015[3] detailed the findings of an investigation into the serious and avoidable failings in maternity and neonatal services at Morecambe Bay NHS Trust, and identified that improvement in maternity safety nationally would usefully address the *whole* maternity system, including workplace behaviour and culture, to improve care and outcomes. Since 2015, multiple maternity improvement reports, initiatives and organizations have all made similar recommendations to use a whole system approach, including personalization of care. 'Better Births'[4] outlined a strategy to implement the findings from the National Maternity Review, through the Maternity Transformation Programme. Further national initiatives, including Each Baby Counts (EBC) and Saving Babies' Lives made recommendations to improve outcomes for women and their babies, with a specific focus on improving intrapartum fetal monitoring.

INTRODUCTION TO NATIONAL INITIATIVES

In this section, we discuss the more significant national initiatives ranging from standard setting, such as the Saving Babies' Lives Care Bundle, to an evaluation of incidents of perinatal mortality and morbidity, to national benchmarking audits such as the National Maternity and Perinatal Audit.

Saving Babies' Lives Care Bundle

First described in the report 'Better Births', the Saving Babies' Lives Care Bundle (SBLCB) (Table 17.1)[5] was published in March 2016 and was designed specifically to reduce the incidence of stillbirth as well as reduce wider adverse neonatal outcomes. The bundle brought together four focused interventions designed to generate improvement, with a fifth element added to version 2 of the package (SBLCBv2).[6] It was proposed that when implemented as a package of recommendations there would be greater benefits achieved at a faster pace than if the improvements were implemented individually.

In particular, it detailed the need for all maternity staff involved in delivering intrapartum care to be annually trained and competency assessed in the interpretation of fetal heart rate monitoring in labour, as well as the implementation of a 'buddy system' to ensure that a second clinician would perform

TABLE 17.1

Saving Babies' Lives Care Bundle[5,6]

Elements of the Saving Babies' Lives Care Bundle
1. Reducing smoking in pregnancy
2. Risk assessment and surveillance of pregnancies for fetal growth restriction
3. Raising awareness of reduced fetal movement
4. Effective fetal monitoring during labour
5. Reducing pre-term birth (SBLCBv2)

an independent review of fetal well-being at regular intervals throughout labour (commonly referred to as 'Fresh Eyes'). In version 2 (2019) of the bundle,[6] a new recommendation was to include the appointment of a fetal monitoring lead midwife for each Trust, with the responsibility of raising standards in their respective trusts, and also to introduce a standardized risk assessment tool to be used at the onset of labour.

Each Baby Counts

Launched in 2014, 'Each Baby Counts' (EBC)[7] was the national quality improvement project developed by the Royal College of Obstetricians and Gynaecologists (RCOG) and the Royal College of Midwives (RCM). Every maternity unit across England reported their data to allow EBC to investigate the critical contributory factors in each case, as well as examine the wider cultural implications of serious incidents and whether the family were involved where possible. Cases eligible for EBC reporting were term births (gestational age >37 weeks) with one of the following features within the first 7 days of life:

- Intrapartum stillbirth
- Early neonatal death (within the first 7 days)
- Severe brain injury sustained during term labour, defined as any baby:
  - Born with grade 3/severe hypoxic ischaemic encephalopathy (HIE) or
  - Who had undergone active therapeutic hypothermia (also known as TH or 'cooling') or
  - Were comatose, in combination with seizures and decreased central tone.

The EBC project collected data continuously from 2015 to 2018[7-9] with the ambition of reducing the incidence of poor intrapartum outcomes by 50% by 2020. Each report also included thematic reviews on key topics emerging from the reviews, including anaesthetic issues, neonatal care, issues with clinical escalation and fetal monitoring.

Despite excellent national participation and analysis of EBC cases with a number of new insights into intrapartum care, the EBC ambition was not achieved, and the final report with recommendations for future practice was published in 2021.[10]

Healthcare Safety Investigation Branch

The Healthcare Safety Investigation Branch (HSIB) maternity investigation programme was established in 2018 with full coverage in England by 2019. The organization investigates all cases of intrapartum stillbirth, early neonatal death or intrapartum brain injury which meets the criteria defined by the Each Baby Counts programme, replacing local/internal reviews. EBC found wide variation in the conduct and quality of local reviews, and that parents and families were not consistently involved in or informed of the investigations that followed harm in many cases. HSIB is dedicated to improving patient safety through independent investigations into NHS-funded care across England, with a move away from organizations investigating their own incidents. The ambition was to standardize serious incident reviews in maternity, to ensure they were conducted to the highest possible standard, with family engagement and involvement throughout to enable all possible learning to be extracted from each case. However, from April 2020, changes were made to the criteria used for opening an investigation due to COVID-19, and this led to the exclusion of cases where babies were cooled but there was no evidence of neurological injury on follow-up testing (e.g., magnetic resonance imaging [MRI]). These cases were directed back to the trust to continue a local investigation. However, if concerns are expressed by the family or the trust in a case where no neurological injury was diagnosed, HSIB will continue to investigate where appropriate. HSIB hosts the single portal of referral for maternity investigations which will then be passed on if relevant to the NHS Resolution Early Notification (EN) Scheme following a triage process.

Once complete, individual HSIB maternity investigation reports are shared with the family, the trust and the healthcare professionals who were involved in the incident. Unlike national reports, the individual maternity investigation reports are not published, but they are used locally as a springboard for improvement.

Furthermore, HSIB has published a number of national reports on key learning themes that have emerged from their case series. To date these have included the following:

- Larger babies
- Summary of themes arising from the HSIB Maternity Programme
- Maternal deaths
- Neonatal collapse alongside skin-to-skin care
- Group B Streptococcus

Early Notification Scheme

In addition to the programmes above that were established to investigate cases of adverse outcomes as well as provide recommendations for improving care, NHS Resolution (the operating name of the NHS Litigation Authority) pioneered the EN Scheme in 2017. The EN scheme was created with the dual objectives of streamlining admission of liability and providing early support to families and staff, as well as dissemination of learning within trusts to prevent spiralling legal costs.[11] Once HSIB has completed its investigations these are referred on to the EN Scheme. The EN scheme then triages these reports, and only in the cases of confirmed intrapartum hypoxic brain injury on MRI a liability investigation is opened.[12] Where the diagnosis of brain injury is more nuanced, the case will be analysed by a clinical review team before progressing (Fig. 17.1).

NHS Resolution is the main indemnifier for clinical negligence for NHS acute trusts in England through its 'Clinical Negligence Scheme for Trusts' (known as CNST). NHS Resolution also provides a maternity incentive scheme (MIS) to incentivize trusts to achieve 10 safety actions curated from contributions by system stakeholders, aiming to improve outcomes for women and their babies. In return for meeting all 10 agreed safety actions, trusts will receive a reduction in their payments to the CNST, which can be a significant cost saving. The MIS incorporates targets including staffing, service-user involvement, training, support from the overall trust safety champions in addition to engagement with HSIB, national improvement initiatives such as SBLCBv2 and the NHS Resolution EN scheme.[13]

NMPA: National Maternity and Perinatal Audit

The National Maternity and Perinatal Audit (NMPA) is led by the Royal College of Obstetricians and Gynaecologists Centre for Quality Improvement and Clinical Audit in partnership with the Royal College of Midwives (RCM), the Royal College of Paediatrics and Child Health (RCPCH) and the London School of Hygiene and Tropical Medicine (LSHTM). The NMPA is commissioned by the Healthcare Quality Improvement Partnership (HQIP) as part of the National Clinical Audit and Patient Outcomes Programme (NCAPOP) on behalf of NHS England, the Welsh Government and the Health Department of the Scottish Government.

This audit aims to evaluate a range of care processes and outcomes, in order to identify good practice and

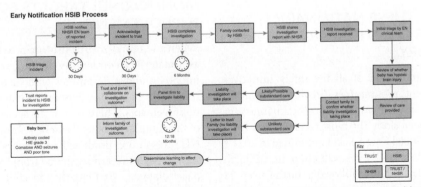

Fig. 17.1 ■ Pathway of investigation from Healthcare Safety Investigation Branch *(HSIB)* to National Health Service Resolution *(NHSR)* Early Notification *(EN)* Scheme.[12] *HIE*, Hypoxic ischaemic encephalopathy.

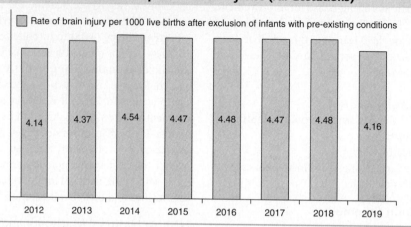

TABLE 17.2

Annual Rate of Intrapartum Brain Injuries (All Gestations)[15]

☐ Rate of brain injury per 1000 live births after exclusion of infants with pre-existing conditions

2012	2013	2014	2015	2016	2017	2018	2019
4.14	4.37	4.54	4.47	4.48	4.47	4.48	4.16

Data from Each Baby Counts represents a specific proportion of intrapartum brain injuries; the numbers in Table 17.3 are limited to intrapartum stillbirths, early neonatal deaths or babies born with hypoxic ischaemic injury from 37 weeks gestation. There is significant morbidity associated with babies born at less than 37 weeks, or due to infection and jaundice at term that is not necessarily captured by Each Baby Counts. Moreover, Each Baby Counts has reported data as absolute numbers rather than a proportion of all births.

areas for improvement in the care of women and babies by NHS maternity services. It uses three lines of investigation to promote this: a survey of maternity care organization nationwide, a continuous prospective clinical audit of key interventions and outcomes and a programme of periodic audits on specific topics.

There have been challenges with timely data, completeness and quality, particularly for England. Completeness of the data for England is anticipated to be higher in future clinical reports, related to anticipated forthcoming improvements in data completeness in the Maternity Services Data Set (MSDS).

IMPACT OF THESE NATIONAL INITIATIVES ON INTRAPARTUM BRAIN INJURY

Despite the introduction of all the safety initiatives and improvement programmes previously detailed, progress in the area of intrapartum brain injury in particular has been slow. The most recent report from the Health and Social Care Select Committee in 2021[14] highlighted a 25% and 29% reduction in stillbirth and neonatal death rates (following births over 24 weeks), respectively, since 2010, however rates of term intrapartum-related neonatal brain injury remain

almost identical to those of 2012, with 4.2 cases per 1000 births.[14] Table 17.2 shows the rate per 1000 live births of all babies born with a brain injury from 2012 to 2019. Birth injuries sustained before labour and birth were excluded. Although there has been a 15% reduction in HIE from 2014 to 2019,[15] the overall rate of change is insufficient to meet the national maternity ambition – to achieve a rate of brain injuries occurring in all gestational ages, during or shortly after labour, of 2.2 per 1000 live births.[14]

INTRAPARTUM FETAL MONITORING: TARGETS FOR IMPROVEMENT

When attempting to establish where to focus our efforts as a maternity community, the various improvement initiatives and programmes with their accompanying reports do shed some light on potential areas to target improvements. There is now an accruing recognition of the complexity of fetal assessment in labour. In 2017 NHS Resolution produced a summary report examining themes and learning shared from 5 years of cerebral palsy claims,[17] particularly the contribution of systemic and human factors to errors with fetal monitoring as one of the key findings from their investigations,

TABLE 17.3			
Babies Reported to Each Baby Counts Over Time[10]			
	2015	2016	2017	2018
Number of babies reported	1136	1123	1130	1145
Rate	1 in 637 (CI 600–675)	1 in 620 (CI 585–658)	1 in 599 (CI 565–636)	1 in 569 (CI 537–604)
Rate per 1000	1.57 (CI 1.48–1.66)	1.61 (CI 1.51–1.71)	1.67 (CI 1.57–1.77)	1.76 (CI 1.66–1.86)

95% confidence intervals presuming a normal distribution.
Each Baby Counts (EBC) highlighted in their initial report that recommendations in healthcare can take up to 17 years to implement and embed successfully[16] and during that time there are potentially thousands of babies and their families who endure preventable and unnecessary harm. The EBC data consistently identified that in approximately 75% of cases different care might have made a difference to the outcome. This highlights that, while disappointing, the lack of progress in brain injury rates is modifiable and can be improved with better care.

not simply individual misinterpretation. In spring 2022 the final Ockenden report was published following an investigation into almost two decades of serious incidents in maternity care at Shrewsbury and Telford NHS Trust.[18] The report detailed 15 immediate and essential actions that should be implemented in all maternity services across England to help improve safety and patient care. It reinforced that system, culture and behaviour-based factors are intricately linked to the improvements in fetal monitoring.

Standardization of Fetal Monitoring Guidelines

Current intrapartum fetal monitoring practice varies widely across the country and even within regions. Currently there are three main CTG classification systems used: National Institute for Health and Care Excellence (NICE),[19] International Federation of Gynaecology and Obstetrics (FIGO)[20] and the so-called Physiological Interpretation.[21] There are also some units who employ a hybrid format, using elements of more than one classification system in their local guidelines (Fig. 17.2). There is enormous potential for confusion and mistakes in this current landscape.

CONTRIBUTORY FACTORS TO ADVERSE OUTCOMES ACCORDING TO EACH BABY COUNTS

Each Baby Counts concluded in 2021, having sadly demonstrated no real shift in the numbers of families suffering the consequences of avoidable intrapartum harm. What they did demonstrate, very clearly for the first time, was the over-simplification of the issue and

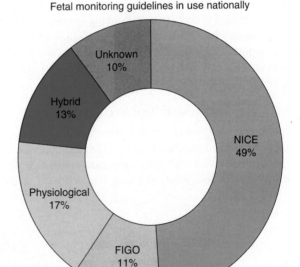

Fetal monitoring guidelines in use nationally

Fig. 17.2 ■ UK fetal monitoring network data on guidelines in use in each Obstetric unit, reproduced with permission from Sarah Blackwell. Data correct as of July 2022, total number of obstetric units 186. The hybrid group includes units who use a combination of fetal monitoring guidelines, namely National Institute for Health and Care Excellence *(NICE)* + Physiological or International Federation of Gynaecology and Obstetrics *(FIGO)* + Physiological.

the complexity of delivering safe intrapartum care. In 74% of the cases they reviewed from 2018, they concluded that different care could have led to a different outcome, and this figure was almost identical to the same statistic from 2015 to 2017 (71% to 76%).[7–10] They also reported repeatedly over consecutive years the same five critical factors identified as contributing to poor outcomes. The five critical contributory factors (excluding neonatal care) are cardiotocography (CTG) and blood sampling, risk recognition, team communication issues, individual human factors and education/training. These top five themes have not changed over previous reports, despite recommendations specifically designed to address them. The focus now needs to move from 'what' needs to change to 'how' that change can be delivered.

Traditionally fetal wellbeing has been synonymous with fetal heart rate changes identified by intermittent auscultation (IA) or continuous CTG. Education and training have therefore focused on the same, albeit with growing recognition of the interplay with human factors in recent years. Looking to other major national reports (HSIB,[22] NHS Resolution,[23] Ockenden reports[18]) the themes for targeting improvement remain strikingly similar and will be explored in more detail as follows.

Lack of Standardized Risk Recognition

It has long been recognized that there is more to intrapartum fetal monitoring than the FHR and other factors are associated with poor neonatal outcomes, e.g., growth restriction, when assessing the wellbeing of a baby in relation to their likely capacity to tolerate the normal physiological stress of labour; otherwise referred to as their 'reserve'. The three main guidelines on fetal heart rate monitoring all agree on the maternal and fetal characteristics where continuous electronic fetal heart rate monitoring should be employed in labour. Emerging evidence suggests that as clinicians we need to be just as mindful of additional features that develop *during* labour. Asma Khalil and colleagues[24] investigated indicators of intrapartum compromise associated with the need for emergency operative birth in 2015 (Fig. 17.3). CTG analysis was a key indicator, but they also identified induction of labour, oxytocin augmentation, intrapartum pyrexia and significant meconium-stained liquor to be associated with emergency operative birth – an intervention used to expedite birth when there is concern for fetal or maternal wellbeing, e.g., an assisted vaginal birth or caesarean section. Another study by Steer et al.[25] of 69 adverse outcomes in the INFANT trial further confirmed the association of induction of labour, oxytocin use, meconium-stained liquor, prolonged labour and pyrexia with subsequent fetal deterioration when present in labour.

The Each Baby Counts Reports have repeatedly highlighted the need for the research community

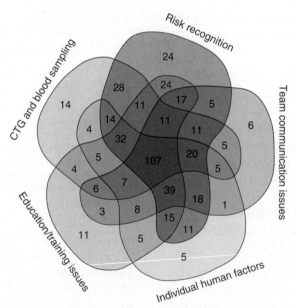

Fig. 17.3 ■ Interrelation of the five most commonly identified themes in the Each Baby Counts final progress report.[10] *CTG,* Cardiotocograph.

to urgently target efforts to establish a more holistic approach to fetal wellbeing in labour, and this was a theme also recognized in the most recent Ockenden final report. The author stated 'Clinicians may miss fetal compromise because current guidelines remain silent on the adverse role played by intrapartum factors, which impair fetal adaptation to the challenges of labour such as fever, chorioamnionitis, meconium…'.[18] Evidence is now accruing that the clinical reasoning applied to the assessment of fetal wellbeing in labour urgently needs updating, to shift the focus from 'is the fetal heart ok?' to 'is the baby ok?'.

Human Factors and Escalation

Following over 400 investigations in the first 20 months of their work, HSIB produced a report summarizing the key patient-safety themes emerging (early recognition of risk, safe intrapartum care, escalation, handovers, larger babies, neonatal collapse alongside skin-to-skin, group B streptococcus and cultural considerations).[22] Delay in risk recognition and escalation of fetal monitoring concerns was a theme that featured in many of their investigations, and is an area intricately linked with human factors or non-technical skills. Human-factor elements of fetal monitoring practice were also examined in more detail in a thematic review of clinical escalation practices in maternity as part of the EBC report in 2019.[9]

The report identified two distinct themes:

1. Poor detection of deterioration and the need to escalate.
2. Poor practices in communicating and responding appropriately.

In relation to detection of deterioration, EBC focused on specific human factors that related to this theme, including cognitive biases, situational awareness and the ability to challenge decisions to name but a few. 'Heuristics' is the name given to the series of mental shortcuts all humans commonly employ when faced with a huge amount of data to analyse and act upon within a short space of time and these can commonly feature in labour ward settings where the workload is mounting alongside a high-stress environment.[26] 'DuPont's Dirty Dozen'[27] recognizes a set of precursors for human error in the aviation industry that is being increasingly utilized in maternity services specifically.[28] The factors of complacency – 'I've seen this before, it was fine then', and normalizing – 'It's a

second-stage CTG', are easily applicable to maternity care and need to be recognized and challenged in order to avoid the harm that can result as a consequence.

Good communication and response to deterioration appropriately require psychological safety, civility and culture with flattened hierarchies and the ability to challenge decisions. A recent report identified that rudeness led to loss of morale for healthcare workers, decreased commitment to work and a reduction in the time spent directly working, leading to a reduction in the quality of their work.[29] The impact of incivility is not confined to the recipient; 20% of witnesses to poor behaviour reported decreases in their performance and 50% of professionals reported being less willing to help others after witnessing uncivil behaviours. Within labour wards, incivility at the point of escalation of deteriorating fetal condition can lead to poor team working and increased likelihood of error. Both the RCOG and the RCM have recognized this and have led many initiatives to improve workplace culture in maternity. A joint workplace behaviour toolkit was made available to their members in 2015 and updated in 2021.[30]

Furthermore, psychological safety is also important within the wider working culture of maternity units. This term refers to staff feeling confident to learn, ask questions, make mistakes or challenge decisions without the fear of reprisal, dismissal or negative consequences, in order to ensure that all members of the clinical team feel encouraged to raise concerns. This principle is discussed in more detail in a recent ethnographic study focusing on features of very safe maternity units,[31] in which the example of senior clinicians highlighting their own mistakes and talking about them openly contributed to a culture of psychological safety, where errors were acknowledged and used for sharing learning instead of being hidden or punished.

Putting all these elements together, it is clear that the role human factors have to play in both individual decision-making as well as the performance and leadership of an overall team cannot be underestimated. Furthermore, these are now considered so vital that mandatory annual training in human factors for all maternity staff is listed as one of the immediate and essential actions in the final Ockenden report.[18]

Team Communication

Detecting deterioration, escalating that concern and in turn responding appropriately, all require clear and effective communication between team members. The use of unequivocal and safety critical language, including unambiguous terminology and closed loop communication, all ensure that the correct message with a clear indication of urgency is received, and that understanding/receipt of the message is confirmed back to the clinician who initiated the communication. The use of structured communication tools, such as SBAR (Situation, Background, Assessment, Recommendation), has been advocated to improve the transfer of critical information between staff at shift changeovers and/or between clinical team members during escalation.

Language and maintenance of escalation momentum during handovers of care are key features of the EBC Learn and Support programme launched in March 2022[32] to help units nationally improve practices critical to safe intrapartum care. Training on structured handover tools during multi-disciplinary training days was also listed as an immediate and essential action from the final Ockenden report.[18]

Education and Training

All practitioners involved in intrapartum care should ensure that they have the knowledge and skills to interpret the CTG and act appropriately, with the aim of providing high-quality, defensible care.

In the UK, issues relating to education and training were considered critical contributory factors to cases of harm in 60% of the investigations where better care could have made a difference to the outcome. Particular issues identified were lack of skill/experience/competence, failure to follow guidelines/locally agreed best practice (the most common factor) and inadequate supervision.[10] These issues have been identified in other European settings. A Swedish study reviewed the outcomes of infants (>33 weeks) born in Stockholm County between 2004 and 2006 and identified substandard care during labour in two thirds of infants with a 5-minute Apgar score of less than 7. The main reasons for the substandard care were related to misinterpretation of the CTG and not acting on a pathological CTG in a timely fashion.[33] These findings were almost exactly replicated in Norway over a similar time period.[34]

More and better training is an almost ubiquitous recommendation, but the evidence supporting training for fetal monitoring is not robust. A systematic review concluded that training can improve CTG competence and clinical practice, but further research is needed to evaluate the type and content of training that is most effective.[35] These findings were further reinforced in a robust, recent systematic review of training for fetal monitoring.[36]

A review of training programmes associated with improvement in clinical outcomes was published in 2009.[37]

Common features of clinically effective training programmes were as follows:

- Multi-professional training
- Training of all staff in an institution
- Training staff locally within the unit in which they work
- Integrating teamwork training with clinical teaching
- Use of high-fidelity simulation models
- Institution-level incentives for training (e.g., reduced hospital insurance premiums)
- Use of self-assessment to directed infrastructural changes

The final Ockenden report published in March 2022 also emphasizes regular, multi-disciplinary, competence-assessed training as vital to the provision of a safe maternity service. Training has been a cornerstone of improvement strategies for decades, but within an often over-stretched service with a chronically short-staffed workforce, it has become increasingly difficult to ensure all staff can access the annual mandatory training needed.

One of the problems with CTG interpretation is that it is difficult and requires a holistic assessment of the women, her labour and appropriate action as well as the fetal heart rate pattern itself. Current UK National guidelines (NICE) standardize the interpretation of intrapartum CTGs, however they are more than 100 pages long,[19,38] which makes them difficult to implement at the coalface of care. Some trusts have adopted techniques to support professionals in practice, e.g., CTG stickers that summarize the guidelines into a simple stick-on format, and these have been successfully introduced into practice with an associated 50% reduction in 5-min Apgar score of less than 7 min and HIE in one UK unit.[39] However it is unlikely to be the sticker itself that improves outcomes. Annual training and support is required to support the use of

CTG stickers and their use should be mandated for all staff whenever a CTG is reviewed and other contrary tools and systems should be stopped.[40] Finally, the use of stickers should be 'policed' using notes audits and the effect on outcomes such as low Apgar scores.

Studies have demonstrated that multi-professional training for CTG interpretation using standardized tools can be effective and have been associated with significant improvements in infants born in poor condition in the UK,[39] the US[41] and Australia.[42] However, there are little data supporting thresholds to pass/fail CTG assessments which have been recommended by SBLCBv2. There is concern about the lack of predictive validity and credentialing strategies, and therefore further research is required before routine adoption or recommendation.

WHERE TO FOCUS OUR EFFORTS?

Collating all the key recommendations from national reports, it is possible to conceptualize an optimal fetal surveillance system, one which would involve an integrated approach as a part of an end-to-end system of care, and include the following:

- Local, multi-professional education and training, particularly to use standardized tools to support best care for intrapartum fetal monitoring.
- Emphasis on a holistic assessment of the woman, her labour and appropriate action as well as the fetal heart rate pattern.
- Tools/techniques for detecting fetal deterioration alongside robust systems to escalate and respond to that concern.
- Awareness of cognitive biases and human factors which may adversely influence detection of deterioration, escalation and performance of the appropriate action/response.
- Psychologically safe maternity units with flattened hierarchies to ensure all feel supported to raise a concern or challenge a decision, and discuss it constructively as a team.
- Emphasis on including women and birth partners as part of the team, to ensure effective communication and supported decision-making throughout.

Designing and implementing such a system is a gargantuan task. The enormous variation in clinical practices, unit dynamics and workforce challenges across the country only confound the difficulty in raising standards nationally. The benefits, however, could be huge. A truly integrated system could translate not only into a reduction in adverse outcomes, but also to better workforce morale and improved retention of staff, with all the consequential benefits they offer. Following nationwide inspections in 2021, the Care Quality Commission (CQC) found that 41% of maternity units were either inadequate or required improvement in patient safety.[43]

Finally, training and quality improvement do not address staffing and estate problems. Midwifery staffing levels are at a crisis point, with 57% reporting in a recent RCM workforce survey that they were considering leaving the profession.[44] More than 80% of obstetric units have gaps in the registrar rota,[45] and 30% of doctors who start training in obstetrics and gynaecology leave before completing the programme.[46] A recent report from the Health and Social Care committee reported that £200–£350 million in investment was needed annually to recruit and retain maternity staff to enable units to function safely and deliver high-quality care.[47] Well-supported staff are more able to deliver safe and compassionate care, and this is crucial to families' experiences of one of the most memorable times of their lives. It is therefore vital that any future work in maternity improvement puts communication and team working with women and birthing people front and centre of any future strategy. Improved birth experiences for women and birth partners through respectful communication and supported decision-making could also pave the way to ensuring the NHS is not only one of the safest healthcare systems in the world in which to have a baby, but also one where both staff and service users feel safe, supported and empowered.

CONCLUSION

Since the national maternity ambition to target improvements in fetal monitoring as a proxy for reducing harm to babies during or shortly after labour, there has been a need for a *whole* system approach. The approach needs to be nationally standardized and led by the professional bodies responsible for delivering and maintaining high standards of midwifery and obstetric care, as well as experts from outside the wider healthcare community who can help align the evidence with human factors, and the behavioural and social sciences that underpin the establishment of thriving multidisciplinary teams working in a culture of safety and respect. The RCOG, the RCM and The Healthcare Improvement Studies (THIS) Institute came together in 2019 to form the Avoiding Brain Injury in Childbirth (ABC) Collaboration. Co-designed with maternity staff, women and their birth partners, there is an ambition to develop a new standardized approach to intrapartum fetal surveillance, utilizing a more holistic perspective of fetal wellbeing. The ABC approach uses fetal heart rate as one of a range of clinical indicators of fetal condition in labour that are tracked hourly to aid in the detection of accumulating risk and fetal deterioration. The project also features guidance and resources on safety culture, team working, escalation practices and communication with both colleagues and women and their birth partners, to improve fetal monitoring as a whole system.

In further recognition of the complexity of delivering safe maternity care, and the necessary investment required in multiple areas of the service, NHS England announced in March 2022 a £127 million boost in funding, with money directed to improving workforce numbers, driving cultural and leadership development from the Local Maternity Systems (LMSs) as well as £45 million to increase the capacity of neonatal units nationally.[48] This funding should contribute to the 'whole system approach' which is much-needed to improve outcomes for babies and their families.

REFERENCES

[1] GOV.UK. New ambition to halve rate of stillbirths and infant deaths. Available: https://www.gov.uk/government/news/new-ambition-to-halve-rate-of-stillbirths-and-infant-deaths. 2015.

[2] Department of Health. Safer maternity care. 2017 Nov.

[3] Dr Bill Kirkup CBE. The report of the Morecambe Bay investigation. 2015 Mar.

[4] NHS England. National maternity review: better births. 2016 Feb.

[5] NHS England. Saving babies' lives care bundle. 2016.

[6] NHS England. Saving babies' lives version 2. 2019 Mar.

[7] Royal College of Obstetricians and Gynaecologists. Each Baby Counts 2015 full report. 2017 Oct.

[8] Royal College of Obstetricians and Gynaecologists. Each Baby Counts 2018 progress report. 2018 Nov.

[9] Royal College of Obstetricians and Gynaecologists. Each Baby Counts 2019 progress report. 2020 Mar.

[10] Royal College of Obstetricians and Gynaecologists. Each Baby Counts 2020 final progress report. 2021 Mar.

[11] NHS Resolution. Available: https://resolution.nhs.uk/services/claims-management/clinical-schemes/clinical-negligence-scheme-for-trusts/early-notification-scheme/.

[12] NHS Resolution. Available: https://resolution.nhs.uk/resources/nhs-resolution-hsib-webinar-on-changes-to-the-early-notification-scheme-june-2021. 2021.

[13] NHS Resolution. Available: https://resolution.nhs.uk/services/claims-management/clinical-schemes/clinical-negligence-scheme-for-trusts/maternity-incentive-scheme/.

[14] Department of Health and Social Care. Safer Maternity Care Progress report 2021. London; 2021.

[15] Gale C, Ougham K, Uthaya S, et al. Brain injury occurring during or soon after birth: annual incidence and rates of brain injuries to monitor progress against the national maternity ambition 2018 and 2019 national data. London; 2021 Jan.

[16] Beauchemin M, Cohn E, Shelton RC. Implementation of clinical practice guidelines in the health care setting. Adv Nurs Sci 2019;42(4):307–24.

[17] NHS Resolution. A summary of: five years of cerebral palsy claims. 2017 Sep.

[18] Ockenden D. Findings, conclusions and essential actions from the independent review of maternity services from the Shrewsbury and Telford Hospital NHS Trust: our final report. 2022 Mar.

[19] NICE. Intrapartum care for healthy women and babies. Clinical guideline [CG190] (updated Feb 2017). 2014 Dec.

[20] Ayres-de-Campos D, Arulkumaran S. FIGO consensus guidelines on intrapartum fetal monitoring: physiology of fetal oxygenation and the main goals of intrapartum fetal monitoring. Int J Gynecol Obstet 2015;131(1):5–8.

[21] Chandrahan E, Evans SA, Krueger D, et al. Available: https://physiological-ctg.com/guideline.html; 2018.

[22] Healthcare Safety Investigation Branch. Summary of themes arising from the healthcare safety investigation Branch maternity programme (April 2018–December 2019). 2020 Mar.

[23] NHS Resolution. A summary of: the Early Notification scheme progress report. 2019 Sep.

[24] Khalil AA, Morales-Rosello J, Morlando M, et al. Is fetal cerebroplacental ratio an independent predictor of intrapartum fetal compromise and neonatal unit admission?. Am J Obstet Gynecol 2015;213(1): 54.e1– 54.e10.

[25] Steer P, Kovar I, McKenzie C, et al. Computerised analysis of intrapartum fetal heart rate patterns and adverse outcomes in the INFANT trial. BJOG An Int J Obstet Gynaecol 2019;126(11):1354–61.

[26] Muoni T. Decision-making, intuition, and the midwife: understanding heuristics. Br J Midwife 2012;20(1):52–6.

[27] https://www.faasafety.gov/files/gslac/library/documents/2012/nov/71574/dirtydozenweb3.pdf.

[28] Nzelu O, Chandraharan E, Pereira S. Human Factors: The Dirty Dozen in CTG misinterpretation. Glob J Reprod Med. 2018;6(2):555683.

[29] Porath C, Pearson C. The price of incivility. Harv Bus Rev. 91(1–2):114–121, 146.

[30] RCOG & RCM. Workplace Behaviour Toolkit. https://www.rcog.org.uk/careers-and-training/starting-your-og-career/workforce/improving-workplace-behaviours/workplace-behaviour-toolkit; 2021.

[31] Liberati EG, Tarrant C, Willars J, et al. How to be a very safe maternity unit: an ethnographic study. Soc Sci Med 2019;223:64–72.

[32] RCOG. Each Baby Counts Learn & Support. Available: https://www.rcog.org.uk/about-us/groups-and-societies/the-rcog-centre-for-quality-improvement-and-clinical-audit/each-baby-counts-learn-support/escalation-toolkit/advice-inform-do-aid/. 2022.

[33] Berglund S, Pettersson H, Cnattingius S, et al. How often is a low Apgar score the result of substandard care during labour? BJOG An Int J Obstet Gynaecol 2010;117(8):968–78.

[34] Andreasen S, Backe B, Jørstad RG, et al. A nationwide descriptive study of obstetric claims for compensation in Norway. Acta Obstet Gynecol Scand 2012;91(10):1191–5.

[35] Pehrson C, Sorensen J, Amer-Wåhlin I. Evaluation and impact of cardiotocography training programmes: a systematic review. BJOG An Int J Obstet Gynaecol 2011;118(8):926–35.

[36] Kelly S, Redmond P, King S, et al. Training in the use of intrapartum electronic fetal monitoring with cardiotocography: systematic review and meta–analysis. BJOG An Int J Obstet Gynaecol. 2021;128(9):1408–19.

[37] Siassakos D, Crofts J, Winter C, et al. The active components of effective training in obstetric emergencies. BJOG An Int J Obstet Gynaecol 2009;116(8):1028–32.

[38] Royal College Obstetricians & Gynaecologists Clinical Effectiveness Unit. The use of electronic fetal monitoring. The use and interpretation of cardiotocography in intrapartum fetal surveillance. Evidence-based clinical guideline number 8. London; 2001.

[39] Draycott T, Sibanda T, Owen L, et al. Does training in obstetric emergencies improve neonatal outcome? BJOG An Int J Obstet Gynaecol 2006;113(2):177–82.

[40] Macrae C, Draycott T. Delivering high reliability in maternity care: in situ simulation as a source of organisational resilience. Saf Sci 2019;117:490–500.

[41] Weiner C, Draycott T. The implementation of PROMPT at the Kansas: Kansas University Medical Centre; 2012.

[42] Victorian Managed Insurance Authority. VicPROMPT Pilot Project Evaluation Report: an evaluation of the VicPROMPT pilot project: a multi-professional obstetric emergencies training program 2010-2011. Melbourne; 2012.

[43] Care Quality Commission. Safety, equity and engagement in maternity services. 2021 Jul.

[44] Royal College of Midwives. RCM members experience survey. 2021.

[45] Kmietowicz Z. Almost nine in 10 obstetric units have unfilled rotas, finds audit. BMJ 2017;358:3855.

[46] RCOG. Obstetrics and Gynaecology. Workforce status report. 2018. p. 2022.

[47] Health and Social Care Committee. The safety of maternity services in England. 2021 Jun.

[48] NHS England. NHS announces £127 million maternity boost for patients and families. Available: https://www.england.nhs.uk/2022/03/nhs-announces-127m-maternity-boost-for-patients-and-families/; 2022.

18 REFLECTIONS AND CONCLUSION

DONALD GIBB ■ SABARATNAM ARULKUMARAN

Our clinical careers began in the first decade of electronic fetal monitoring (EFM). Randomized trials and evidence-based medicine were in their infancy. Fetal scalp blood sampling had been introduced in advance of EFM in the early 1970s. Neither were based on evidence-based medicine, but there was an assumption that technology would produce results. Unfortunately, we have been disappointed. We have not seen the improvements in outcome that we had hoped for. This is a time for reflection.

No technique should be introduced without structured training and education. However, a need was seen and quite rapidly the technology was introduced in industrialized countries. Maternal and perinatal outcomes were improving in these countries, but this was likely to be due to improving social conditions, better nutrition and fertility control as well as improved care. To what degree EFM was contributing to this was unclear. Several trials suggested that EFM was not having a great effect. Although trial structure and methodology may be criticized the message was disconcerting. After extensive exposure to the use of EFM in Kandang Kerbau Hospital, Singapore, we decided to write this handbook and introduce cardiotocograph (CTG) education seminars. We published the first edition in 1992. For 15 years we pursued a vigorous programme of education internationally. This could never be enough and was beyond the scope of a few individuals. We hope it inspired others to take up the cause.

Recent years have seen various initiatives by UK and international bodies to address these issues. They have been able to illustrate a poor state of affairs but with little progress or improvement. It seems a wider perspective is required. The reports we have seen of poor care refer to not only misunderstandings of the CTG but also of systems failures. Obstetrics is unique requiring close team working with midwives. Educational initiatives around pregnancy care should involve doctors and midwives. It is interesting and hopefully symbolic that the Royal College of Obstetricians and Gynaecologists (RCOG) and Royal College of Midwives (RCM) now operate from the same new building.

There are critical issues that need to be addressed as suggested by the reports produced by Kirkup and Ockenden. Sadly, more adverse publicity is being generated from other maternity units. We need to be radical in our practice reviews. A good working environment is essential. Staffing shortage and underfunding need to be corrected. Bullying both between midwives and between midwives and doctors must be rooted out. A high level of interdisciplinary working between doctors, midwives, neonatal staff and anaesthetic colleagues must be promoted. This is the important system context in which education and training lie. There is no doubt that broad-based training in fetal monitoring and clinical situations is important, but the context must be addressed. There is a huge task to undertake, but faced with parents unhappy with outcomes and relentless escalation of litigation and its costs, it cannot be avoided.

There has been a lot of discussion about guidelines and the fact that there are currently three sets available (see Chapter 17). This should not be necessary and we have chosen to focus on the International Federation of Obstetrics and Gynaecology (FIGO) Guidelines (see Chapter 6). All of these guidelines are based on physiological and pathophysiological principles as detailed in Chapter 5. International agreement is important.

The National Institute for Health and Care Excellence (NICE) guidelines are too conditional and detailed in the tables of categories and management. They are difficult to memorize. We also disagree with the de-emphasis on the admission CTG in the NICE guidelines. In our experience the admission CTG can sometimes produce a surprising and unexpected finding, even in a low-risk case.

After long experience in the clinical scenario and, sadly, experience with case review and the law court courts, we would highlight a few issues.

It should always be ensured that what is being recorded is the fetal heart and not the maternal pulse. This is particularly a hazard in the late first stage and second stage of labour. If the nature of the trace changes usually to a more 'normal' rate it may be the maternal pulse. A very abnormal fetal heart rate may be hidden or even absent. This issue should be explained to every junior obstetrician and every junior midwife as one of the first lessons in fetal assessment. It is a catastrophe to have to explain to the parents that the baby was seriously compromised or dead when it was thought to be healthy. We ourselves were not aware of this in the early part of our careers.

As highlighted by Professor Steer (see Chapter 16) the misuse of syntocinon contributes to many sad cases in litigation. Continuing a syntocinon infusion at the same or greater rate in spite of an abnormal CTG, meconium-stained amniotic fluid and good progress in labour is a common avoidable error. This may also drive the head lower into the pelvis, culminating in a difficult Caesarean section at full dilatation. This is a serious maternal risk and has only been recognized as so in recent years.

One or more risk factors may be observed in the same case. Known risk factors are small baby, induction of labour, abnormal CTG, use of syntocinon, fetal scalp blood sampling. Missing to recognise the cumulating risks lead to poor outcome due to human factor. Fetal scalp blood sampling should only be done when approved by senior staff. Referral should be made to Chapter 14: when not to perform a fetal scalp blood sample. A thorough understanding of CTG interpretation should reduce the need for fetal scalp blood sampling.

Human factors will become more of a focus as suggested in Chapter 17. A happy and motivated team is crucial. Proper funding, adequate staffing, education and leadership are all essential. A duty of candour when things go wrong is a 'must'. We hope the Avoiding Brain Injury in Child-birth (ABC) initiative will bear fruit.

We trust that handing over of practical knowledge to a new generation of clinicians would improve the quality of care. Great care in childbirth is an essential part of a civilized society. Empathy and humanity are the cornerstones.

We thank all the contributors. We have introduced and integrated new authors, which we hope will rejuvenate and contribute to the continuing relevance of this handbook.

INDEX

Note: Page numbers followed by *b* indicates boxes, *f* indicates figures, and *t* indicates tables.